the prediabetes detox

a whole-body program *to* balance your blood sugar, increase energy, *and* reduce sugar cravings

SARAH CIMPERMAN, ND

New Harbinger Publications, Inc.

Publisher's Note

This publication is designed to provide accurate and authoritative information in regard to the subject matter covered. It is sold with the understanding that the publisher is not engaged in rendering psychological, financial, legal, or other professional services. If expert assistance or counseling is needed, the services of a competent professional should be sought.

Distributed in Canada by Raincoast Books

Copyright © 2013 by Sarah Cimperman
        New Harbinger Publications, Inc.
        5674 Shattuck Avenue
        Oakland, CA 94609
        www.newharbinger.com

Cover design by Amy Shoup
Text design by Michele Waters-Kermes
Acquired by Jess O'Brien
Edited by Brady Kahn

Library of Congress Cataloging-in-Publication Data on file

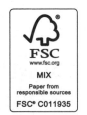

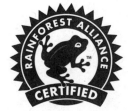

Printed in the United States of America

FSC
www.fsc.org
MIX
Paper from responsible sources
FSC® C011935

15   14   13

10   9   8   7   6   5   4   3   2   1   First printing

"A fascinating book by Sarah Cimperman! Diabetes is certainly an epidemic of mass proportions that hasn't been properly prevented. She provides sound evidence to support why detoxing and using nutritional supplements can help ward off harmful complications of diabetes. Her book guides you through easy-to-follow steps to improved health."

—**Jessica Black, ND**, best-selling author of *The Anti-Inflammation Diet and Recipe Book*

"I'm a big believer in healthy eating and detoxification, and I agree with what Cimperman has to say about it in her new book, *The Prediabetes Detox*. I like her emphasis on healthy fats, and not just from fish, but also avocados, raw nuts, and coconuts. Fat has gotten a lot of bad press, but healthy fats support a healthy brain, beautify the skin, and are building blocks for vital hormones."

—**Eric R. Braverman, MD**, director of the PATH Medical Center and PATH Foundation

"Cimperman has written a reliable, informative, and easy-to-follow guide for managing prediabetes. It is a beautifully written work that provides readers with a practical program of action and sound advice. *The Prediabetes Detox* is a must-read for anyone interested in improving their health and preventing diabetes. I am pleased to recommend this book."

—**Marianne Marchese, ND**, author of *8 Weeks to Women's Wellness*

"I diagnose prediabetes regularly in my practice and usually have fifteen minutes to explain lifestyle changes. I welcome Cimperman's book because it gives detailed recommendations on how to make these lifestyle changes. Cimperman uses evidence-based advice that initially may seem difficult but ultimately empowers patients to take charge of their health by making life long changes that will truly reverse disease and improve overall well-being."

—**Joyce Qaqundah MD**, family medicine physician, San Diego

This book is dedicated to my patients,
who inspire me every day.

Contents

Recipes

Foreword

Our nation is in the middle of a serious epidemic, and I am not referring to whichever virulent flu is going around. Nor am I referring to cancer or heart disease. I am referring to elevated blood sugar (prediabetes and type 2 diabetes). As with most of our chronic illnesses, this one is clearly linked to lifestyle factors—what we do or do not put into our mouths and what we do or do not do with our bodies. The last estimate of annual sugar intake by the average US resident was right around one hundred pounds per year. Next time you are at the grocery store, look at the five-pound bags of sugar and think about having twenty of them in your pantry and having to consume them all within twelve months. You probably wouldn't even consider consuming that much white sugar right out of the bag, but the average American does eat that much, partly because sugar is hidden in so many places you wouldn't expect. Little wonder many people do not feel well!

Perhaps you, like most people, know you should eat more healthily but fear you'd be doomed to eating food that is boring or tastes bad. Personally, I would choose to give up a few of the best-tasting foods in exchange for a life without all of the health complaints I have heard from my patients over the last thirty years. In fact, it is primarily from watching what has happened with my patients that I have become such a proponent of good nutrition and less-toxic living. The more patient stories I heard, the bigger my backyard organic garden grew, the less toxic our indoor air became, and the more my sugar intake shrank. And I've been pleased to discover that healthy food can be delicious and convenient.

If you'd like to live well no matter what your age, this is the book for you. Dr. Cimperman will take you on a fantastic journey through your body. She will explain how your body responds differently to the various carbohydrates and fats in your diet. You will learn the difference between foods that cause inflammation (which underlies chronic pain, among other problems) and foods that reduce inflammation. You will also learn about common environmental toxicants that can sap your energy and contribute to fatigue, obesity, and blood-sugar problems. She will then show you simple ways to reduce your daily exposure to these toxicants and help your body get rid of those that are already present.

When I tell patients to clear various foods from their diet, like white sugar and white flour products, they sometimes ask what else there is to eat. Dr. Cimperman expertly handles this issue by discussing the foods that you can add to your diet to optimize your health. This should help you to expand your food-selection horizons, which will make it much easier to eat a healthier diet that will delight your taste buds as well as your cells. She then expertly covers the basics of nutritional supplementation that will help to seal the deal on vibrant health. I can say with absolute certainty that the diet and supplement plan contained in this book will help you lead a better life. Here's to your health!

—Walter Crinnion, ND

Acknowledgments

I'd like to thank Wendy Millstine, acquisitions editor at New Harbinger, for her enthusiasm for this project and her expertise during the development of the proposal for this book.

I'd like to thank my husband, Bruno, for giving me the time and space I needed to write this book and also for tearing me away from my work occasionally to whisk me off on amazing adventures. Thank you for always reminding me that work and play are equally important ingredients in a happy and healthy life.

I'd like to thank my mother, Janis, the epitome of a strong and successful role model, and my father, Dwight, the world's most supportive dad.

I'd like to thank my friend and colleague Dr. Noreen Lalani, who encouraged me to write my first article; Mary Arsenault, publisher of *Wisdom* magazine, who published my first article and gave me my first column; and my friend Juliah Lindsey, who encouraged me to write my first blog. I'd like to thank my friend Maya Camou, who is also my loudest cheerleader, for her tough love and endless encouragement.

And I'd like to thank all of the women who have shared my kitchen, invited me into theirs, and inspired my cooking. Among them: my mother Janis Cimperman, my grandmother Lucille Lundstrom, Janna Graham, who taught me to love making meals from scratch (and Mollie Katzen, whose *Enchanted Broccoli Forest* cookbook was our bible); Juliah Lindsey, who has been known to add fresh ginger to everything (literally) and fish sauce to anything (even yogurt-based vinaigrettes with surprisingly good results); Dr.

Michelle Qaqundah, who showed me how easy and fun it is to make sushi at home; Dr. Keely Killpack, campfire gourmet, who has been known to make the most delicious meals in the middle of the Oregon wilderness; my sister Jennifer Cimperman, who is one of the most creative and adventurous cooks I know; my mother-in-law, Méranie Lamarre, who taught me to cook fish and seafood (among many other things) on the beautiful island of Martinique; and my husband's late grandmother, Jeanine Lamarre, who taught me the art of French cuisine in her lively kitchen in the French countryside.

I'd also like to acknowledge Dr. Walter Crinnion, who taught me environmental medicine in medical school, and Hannah Reich, for her words of wisdom during the publishing process. And I'd like to thank Jess Beebe, Jess O'Brien, Amy Shoup, Heather Garnos, Michele-Waters Kermes, and Angela Autry Gordon of New Harbinger Publications, along with copyeditor Brady Kahn and proofreader Elizabeth Kennedy, for their valuable input on this book.

Introduction

If you're one of the seventy-nine million people in the United States living with prediabetes, you've likely been counseled to change your diet and to exercise more. There's no doubt that diet and exercise are crucial, and you'll want to make a serious commitment to both. But there are other powerful steps you can take to improve your health. Studies show that toxic chemicals in our food and water can cause changes in the body that promote the development of diabetes. These *diabetogens* include pesticides, chemicals in nonstick cookware and plastic food and beverage containers, industrial pollutants absorbed by some of the plants and animals in our diet, and chemicals found in our drinking water.

Since 1999 the National Center for Health Statistics, part of the Centers for Disease Control and Prevention, has measured chemicals in the blood and urine of people taking part in the National Health and Nutrition Examination Survey. The most recent report found diabetogenic chemicals in every single sample (CDC 2013). That's right: 100 percent of the 2,500 people studied tested positive for toxins that are found in food and have been shown to increase the risk of diabetes.

We may not be able to avoid all of the toxins in our diet, but we can take steps to minimize our exposure and remove them from our bodies through detoxification. Detox is especially important for people with prediabetes, as it's an essential part of reversing the condition. The prediabetes detox program that this book offers is a combination of a healthy diet, regular exercise, supplements, and activities that help your body eliminate toxins. I've designed it with these goals in mind:

- Reduce the intake of harmful chemicals in food and water.

- Mobilize and excrete the toxins already stored inside the body.

- Burn fat instead of accumulate fat.

- Normalize blood sugar and insulin levels.

These goals may sound lofty, but they are entirely achievable. Changing your diet and lifestyle really can change the way your body uses energy, stores energy, and reacts to chemicals in the environment.

As a naturopathic doctor, I have a holistic approach to medicine. (You can learn more about naturopathic medicine at www.prediab tesdetox.com.) Instead of treating symptoms, it's my goal to identify and address the underlying causes of illness using the most natural and least toxic therapies available. Detoxification is one of these therapies. Along with regular exercise and permanent changes in diet and lifestyle, detox is one of the most powerful tools we can use to improve our health. It gives us a break from environmental stressors and replenishes us with the good food, good exercise, and good sleep our bodies need to repair, rebuild, regenerate, and rejuvenate. Detoxification is like a tune-up for the whole body.

I've been using detox in my practice for more than a decade, and I've found it to be particularly effective for reversing prediabetes. After my patients complete the program, they report more energy, better sleep, improved moods, weight loss, fat loss, and greater hunger control. Their bowels work better, their skin is clearer, and their focus is sharper. Their tastes have changed, and their cravings for sugar and carbohydrate-rich foods have been replaced with a true desire to eat healthy, nourishing food. They are inspired to exercise because they know how much better they feel when it's a regular part of their routine. They feel a renewed sense of vitality and get sick less often. Minor complaints they had before detoxification, like indigestion, bloating, and puffiness, often resolve spontaneously. And as an added bonus for normalizing blood sugar and insulin levels, these patients reduce their risk of heart disease, stroke, obesity, dementia, and cancer. They don't just live longer; they live better. You can do it too.

This book will be your guide. Chapter 1 introduces prediabetes: what it is, why it happens, and how to find out if you have it. It will also share with you the ten most dangerous foods for people with prediabetes. Chapter 2 covers detoxification: what it really means, what it accomplishes, what to expect, and how to prepare. Most people can follow this program safely at home, but it's not right for everyone, so this chapter also will cover who should not detox and who should see their doctor before they start. Chapter 3 introduces the prediabetes detox diet, which is naturally gluten-free and appropriate for individuals with celiac disease and wheat or gluten intolerances. This chapter gives general guidelines, as well as specific lists of foods and beverages, so it will be easy to understand what to consume and what to avoid. Chapter 4 discusses the supplements I recommend for detoxification and reversing prediabetes, and chapter 5 discusses the importance of exercise, sleep, saunas, stress management, and other lifestyle interventions for reversing prediabetes. Chapter 6 talks about nonfood sources of toxins, or, more specifically, which chemicals in your environment have been shown to increase the risk of diabetes, where they're found, and how to minimize your exposure. Chapter 7 discusses what to do when the detox is over and gives you a long-term plan for reversing prediabetes permanently and maintaining optimal health. Chapter 8 will help you put my dietary recommendations into practice. It will review the top twelve detox foods and give you recipes to help you get started. And at the end of the book, you'll find a list of references in case you want to learn more about the science behind the prediabetes detox program.

On the www.prediabetesdetox.com website, you'll find more information and support:

- A daily detox checklist to help you keep track of the different components of this program

- More detox-friendly recipes

- Sample menus for omnivores, vegetarians, and those following a dairy-free diet

- Shopping lists
- A chart to help you track the foods you'll reintroduce into your diet after detoxification
- Two examples of weeklong exercise regimens that fit the detox guidelines
- More relaxation exercises
- Instructions for creating some homemade personal products
- Recommended reading and a list of resources to help you find all the things I talk about in this book
- More information about naturopathic medicine

This isn't just another program. It's the beginning of a new chapter in your life. The prediabetes detox program will teach you how to take control of your health, lower your blood sugar and insulin levels, and reverse prediabetes. You'll also learn how easy it is to eat well and how simple it can be to make delicious and healthy meals that your whole family will enjoy.

It's time to get started.

chapter 1
Prediabetes 101

Prediabetes is a worldwide epidemic.. In the United States alone, it affects one in three adults. It's a dangerous condition that increases the risk of five of the seven leading causes of US deaths: diabetes, heart disease, stroke, Alzheimer's disease, and cancer. Prediabetes also increases the risk of debilitating conditions like blindness, amputation, kidney problems, and immobility, as well as dependence on caregivers. The good news is that prediabetes is reversible. It's a state of imbalance, not permanent dysfunction, and a signal that your body needs a tune-up, now.

The best cure for prediabetes is not prescription medication. While pharmaceutical drugs can be lifesavers in certain circumstances, they're not always necessary, and when it comes to reversing prediabetes, they aren't the best place to start. A landmark study published in the prestigious *New England Journal of Medicine* compared the effects of diabetes drug Glucophage (metformin) to diet and lifestyle changes (Knowler et al. 2002). Twenty-seven medical centers around the country and more than three thousand people with prediabetes were randomly split into three treatment groups. One group exercised for two and a half hours each week and received sixteen one-on-one lessons focusing on diet, exercise, and behavior modification during the first twenty-four weeks; they also participated in subsequent monthly individual and group sessions designed to reinforce these lifestyle changes. Another group took Glucophage, and the third group took placebo pills. Participants in these two groups also received written information about a healthy lifestyle and twenty to thirty minutes of individual counseling once each year.

After three years, participants in the intensive lifestyle intervention group reduced their risk of diabetes by 58 percent (with adults above the age of sixty reducing their risk by 71 percent) compared to participants receiving the placebo, regardless of their gender or ethnicity, while the group taking Glucophage reduced their risk by only 31 percent. (Glucophage was most effective for people at least sixty pounds overweight and least effective in adults over the age of forty-five.) Benefits of the intensive lifestyle interventions were still apparent a decade later. Ten years after the initial study, researchers found that people in the lifestyle group still had a 43 percent lower risk of developing diabetes (adults aged sixty and older had a 49 percent lower risk) while those taking Glucophage had only an 18 percent lower risk.

Another clinical trial compared standard conventional care to a combination of conventional care and naturopathic care (Bradley et al. 2012). Licensed naturopathic doctors are trained as primary care physicians and experts in natural therapies, including diet, exercise, lifestyle counseling, and detoxification. They have a holistic philosophy and a comprehensive approach. In this study, researchers followed adults with type 2 diabetes for one year and compared them to people of similar age and gender who were taking similar diabetes medications and had similar baseline levels of hemoglobin A1C. The participants given combination care received up to eight visits with licensed naturopathic physicians over a one-year period. At the end of the study, they reduced their hemoglobin A1C levels by 0.90 percent while those receiving conventional care saw reductions of only 0.51 percent. The people working with naturopathic doctors also lowered their blood sugar (no changes in blood sugar were observed in those receiving conventional care only) and saw greater improvements in motivation, mood, diet changes, and physical activity.

Now it's your turn to lower your blood sugar and reverse prediabetes using a comprehensive naturopathic approach. But first, this chapter will give you some basic facts about prediabetes and the two major underlying factors: diet and inflammation.

Prediabetes Defined

Prediabetes means having high blood sugar and/or insulin levels. It increases your risk for developing diabetes and other chronic illnesses like cardiovascular disease, dementia, and cancer. Prediabetes is a warning sign that your body is having problems converting sugar from food into energy. If you have prediabetes, your blood sugar levels are above average but not yet high enough to be classified as type 2 diabetes. (Type 1 diabetes is an autoimmune condition where the body attacks insulin-making cells in the pancreas.) When prediabetes is left untreated, most people will develop type 2 diabetes within ten years (NIDDK 2012).

The Centers for Disease Control and Prevention estimate that there are seven million people in the United States with prediabetes who don't even know they have it (CDC 2013). This isn't surprising, because most of the time, there aren't any symptoms. When symptoms do appear, they can include fatigue, an increase in appetite, cravings for sugar and other carbohydrate-rich foods, fat accumulation, and a condition called *acanthosis nigricans*, areas of darker, thicker skin around body creases in the neck, armpits, elbows, knuckles, hips, knees, and toes. Excessive thirst, excessive hunger, excessive urination, and blurred vision can also occur, but these signs are more commonly associated with the onset of type 2 diabetes.

Even if you don't have any symptoms and can't feel prediabetes, damage is still being done. High levels of blood sugar cause inflammation, genetic mutations (Lee and Cerami 1987), cellular damage, and premature aging (Danby 2010). Cells lining blood vessels are particularly vulnerable to damage from high levels of blood sugar. Over time, damaged blood vessels cause problems with the eyes, kidneys, nerves, and heart. High levels of blood sugar also promote the growth of several major cancers, and even small elevations (blood sugar levels above 125 milligrams per deciliter) greatly increase the risk of developing cancer and dying from cancer, according to a study published in the *Journal of the American Medical Association* (Jee et al. 2005).

Diagnostic Tests

It may be difficult for you to tell if you have prediabetes, but your doctor will be able to tell. These are the tests I recommend.

Fasting Plasma Glucose Test

A fasting plasma glucose test measures levels of blood sugar after an overnight or eight-hour fast. Ideally, a blood sample is taken first thing in the morning before breakfast. Fasting glucose levels above eighty-seven milligrams per deciliter are associated with an increased risk of diabetes, and people with the lowest risk have levels below eighty-one milligrams per deciliter (Tirosh et al. 2005).

A fasting plasma glucose test is usually one of the routine screening tests that doctors perform on an annual basis when they order blood work. It's important information, but it isn't the best test for prediabetes, because in the earliest stages, insulin levels often rise first, long before fasting blood sugar levels go up. So it's possible to have a normal fasting blood sugar level and to have prediabetes. If you're having symptoms like weight gain or food cravings, or if your fasting blood glucose level is higher than eighty milligrams per deciliter, you should take the insulin glucose tolerance test and the hemoglobin A1C test.

Insulin Glucose Tolerance Test

The insulin glucose tolerance test measures your body's response to eating sugar. Like the fasting plasma glucose test, it must be done after an overnight or eight-hour fast. For this test, you will be asked to drink a beverage containing seventy-five grams of glucose and to give two blood samples, one before you drink the glucose which confirms your fasting glucose level and another two hours afterward, which measures your *postprandial* glucose level (the amount of sugar in your blood after eating a meal or, in this case, after consuming a glucose drink). Glucose levels should not exceed 120 milligrams per deciliter two hours postprandially. Insulin levels should be less than five microunits per milliliter when fasting and less than thirty postprandially. If your levels exceed these numbers, you have prediabetes.

It's common for doctors to order a tolerance test for glucose only, which is called a glucose tolerance test. But because you could have normal glucose levels and elevated insulin levels, be sure that your doctor is ordering tests for both glucose and insulin.

Hemoglobin A1C Test

The hemoglobin A1C test is also known as the *glycosylated hemoglobin test*. It measures blood sugar attached to hemoglobin, the red pigment in blood cells that transports oxygen around the body. Blood sugar attaches to hemoglobin in proportion to its concentration in the blood, so the higher your blood sugar levels, the more sugar will be attached to your hemoglobin. A blood sample is required for this test, but fasting isn't necessary. Ideally, your hemoglobin A1C level should be less than 5.7 percent. Percentages between 5.7 and 6.4 indicate prediabetes, and two separate test results of 6.5 percent or higher indicate diabetes.

The hemoglobin A1C test has a big advantage over the fasting plasma glucose test, for it reflects blood sugar levels over an extended period of time, not just on one given day. Red blood cells circulate for up to 120 days, so your hemoglobin A1C level gives your doctor a good idea of how high your average blood sugar levels have been over the past few months. However, this test may not be accurate for certain people, including pregnant women, anyone without a spleen, anyone who has had recent blood loss or a blood transfusion, and anyone with anemia, kidney or liver disease, alcohol toxicity, lead toxicity, or uncommon forms of hemoglobin. If this list includes you, your doctor will have to rely on the insulin glucose tolerance test to determine if you have prediabetes.

Vitamin D Test

Because low levels of vitamin D can be an underlying factor risk factor for prediabetes, I also recommend testing 25-hydroxyvitamin D (also known as 25(OH)D3). Studies show that low vitamin D is associated with high fasting plasma glucose levels, regardless of age, gender, ethnicity, body mass index, physical activity, or socioeconomic status (Reis et al. 2009). It's a simple blood test, and it doesn't require fasting. Levels between thirty and eighty nanograms per milliliter are considered normal.

Carbohydrate Metabolism

To understand where blood sugar comes from and how it can get too high, you need to have a basic understanding of how our bodies process food and use energy. In general, all foods are made up of *macronutrients* and *micronutrients*. Macronutrients are present in large amounts and include carbohydrates, fats, and protein. Micronutrients are present in small amounts and include vitamins, minerals, and antioxidants. Foods that come from animals, including meat, eggs, and dairy products, are composed primarily of fat and protein, with little or no carbohydrates. Foods that come from plants, such as fruits and vegetables, are composed primarily of carbohydrates with small amounts of fat and protein. (Certain plant foods contain higher concentrations of protein, like beans and nuts, or higher concentrations of fat, like olives and avocados.) Plant foods also contain fiber, a special form of carbohydrates that humans can't digest, which helps move food through our intestines.

Carbohydrates are made up of sugar molecules, which are made up of water and carbon (a natural element you may remember from the periodic table in chemistry class). Sometimes sugar molecules exist alone, and other times they are linked together in chains. Depending on the number of sugars in each chain, they are categorized as *simple* or *complex*. Simple carbohydrates contain only one or two sugar molecules, while complex carbohydrates contain at least three and sometimes thousands of sugar molecules. Simple carbohydrates are found in processed foods, sweets, and starches like baked goods, pasta, rice, and potatoes. Complex carbohydrates are found in whole foods like vegetables, beans, and nuts.

Because our bodies can't absorb long chains of sugar molecules, they must be digested, or broken down, into single sugars first. Carbohydrate digestion starts in the mouth, when chewing stimulates our salivary glands to secrete enzymes that break apart sugar chains. This process continues in the stomach and concludes in the small intestine where single sugars are absorbed into the bloodstream. Whenever we eat carbohydrates and whenever our taste buds detect something sweet, even in the absence of carbohydrates (as when we ingest artificial sweeteners), our pancreas releases the hormone insulin. Cells need insulin to absorb sugar from the blood. Insulin acts like a key, opening doors to cells and allowing sugar inside where it can be burned for energy. Without insulin, cells can't absorb sugar from the blood. Without sugar, cells can't produce the energy they need to function.

The amount of insulin released is proportional to the amount of sugar in the blood—so low levels of blood sugar trigger low levels of insulin, and high levels of blood sugar trigger high levels of insulin—and the amount of sugar in the blood is determined by the foods that we eat. Carbohydrates in whole foods are long chains of sugars that are chemically bonded to fat, protein, fiber, and micronutrients. It takes several hours and several different enzymes to break these foods down and separate the sugars before we can absorb them. Because the digestion of complex carbohydrates is a slow process, sugars are absorbed slowly into the body, and blood sugar and insulin levels rise slowly in response. These can be called *slow carbohydrates*. The single sugars in simple carbohydrates don't require digestion, because they are not chemically bound to other sugars, fat, protein, fiber, or micronutrients. They are absorbed immediately and flood the body with sugar. Insulin levels skyrocket in response. These can be called *fast carbohydrates*.

High levels of insulin send a message to the brain that our immediate energy needs have been met. In response, the body stores excess sugar as an energy reserve for future use, in case food were to become scarce. Some sugar is turned into a compound called *glycogen* and stored in liver and muscle cells for short-term use in case we need it quickly, but most excess sugar is converted into fat for long-term storage. That's right: the body turns sugar into fat when insulin levels are high. High insulin levels also trap fatty acids inside fat cells, so it is impossible to burn fat for energy. When blood sugar levels are high, you will always accumulate fat. But when blood sugar and insulin levels are low, the body turns fat back into sugar to be used for energy. So whether our bodies burn fat or accumulate fat depends on what kind of carbohydrates we eat and how much of them we eat at one time.

When blood sugar and insulin levels are too high for too long, our cells start to resist. They ignore the effects of insulin and become less effective at taking up sugar from the blood. Insulin resistance causes sugar to build up in the blood and, as a result, the pancreas secretes even more insulin in an effort to clear it. Eventually, the pancreas may not be able to make enough insulin to meet the body's needs. If there isn't enough insulin or if cells don't respond to it normally, the cells starve because they can't absorb enough sugar to generate adequate energy. Starving cells trigger hunger and cravings for fast carbs because fast carbs are the quickest source of energy and because raising blood sugar levels quickly is the fastest way to lower high insulin levels. However, eating more sugar only perpetuates the cycle and makes matters worse. When the body develops insulin resistance and/or loses the ability to produce enough insulin to meet its needs, prediabetes turns into type 2 diabetes.

Fast Carbs

For people with prediabetes, fast carbs are the most dangerous foods. They are quickly digested and rapidly absorbed into the bloodstream, flooding the body with sugar and prompting the release of large amounts of insulin, which can trigger weight gain, food cravings, and fatigue. Here are the top ten worst offenders:

- Natural and artificial sweeteners
- Baked goods
- Pasta
- Breakfast cereals

- Whole grains

- Starchy vegetables

- Starchy fruits

- Processed fruit

- Soft drinks

- Milk

The foods on this list are worth exploring further.

Sweeteners

The general category of sweeteners includes all forms of sugar: white, brown, cane, beet, date, grape, granulated, powdered, and even raw. It includes evaporated cane juice and liquid sweeteners like agave nectar, agave syrup, maple syrup, honey, rice syrup, brown rice syrup, barley malt syrup, corn syrup, high fructose corn syrup, carob syrup, caramel, molasses, sorghum, fruit juice, and fruit juice concentrate. It includes sugar alcohols, like mannitol, sorbitol, and xylitol, and sugar additives, like dextrose, maltose, sucrose, lactose, galactose, glucose, and fructose.

This category also includes all artificial sweeteners like saccharin (sold as Sweet'N Low), aspartame (sold as Equal or NutraSweet), sucralose (sold as Splenda), neotame (chemically similar to aspartame), and acesulfame potassium (found in sodas and baked goods). Artificial sweeteners are often recommended for people with prediabetes and diabetes because they don't raise blood sugar levels, but because they taste sweet, they do raise insulin levels, promoting hunger and fat accumulation. Remember that the sensation of sweet flavors on your tongue is enough to prompt your pancreas to secrete insulin. Studies show that artificial sweeteners have the same effect as sugar on insulin levels (Liang et al. 1987). Artificial sweeteners also make your taste buds accustomed to very sweet flavors, and they can compromise the body's natural detoxification mechanisms. Researchers in North Carolina found that Splenda altered the body's ability to excrete medications, changed the pH of the gastrointestinal tract, and lowered levels of beneficial bacteria in the intestines

(Abou-Donia et al. 2008). Having healthy populations of beneficial bacteria is especially important for detoxification and for reversing prediabetes.

There is one exception to this rule: stevia. It's an herbaceous plant from South America with naturally sweet-tasting leaves, thanks to a compound called stevioside. Animal studies show that stevia can improve insulin sensitivity (Chang et al. 2005), and human studies show that it can lower levels of glucose and insulin (Gregersen et al. 2004). Randomized, double-blind, placebo-controlled, long-term studies show that stevia has an excellent safety record and is well tolerated in people with and without diabetes (Barriocanal et al. 2008). It's better to avoid sweets completely, but for those who can't live without something sweet, the best choice is small amounts of pure stevia, up to one gram (the amount used in studies) per day. Stevia comes in both powder and liquid forms, and some products have a bitter aftertaste. Always read the label to make sure there are no other ingredients and to determine the serving size equal to one gram.

Processed Grains

This category includes white rice and all foods made with flour, such as breads, pastries, pasta, and cereals, whether or not they contain gluten, whether they're made with white flour or whole-grain flour, and whether they are derived from wheat or alternative grains like spelt, rice, or quinoa. This includes bread, rolls, buns, toast, toaster pastries, breadsticks, bread crumbs, baguettes, bagels, croissants, muffins, scones, English muffins, crumpets, biscuits, pita bread, pretzels, crackers, pizza, quiche, pies, tarts, cakes, cupcakes, cookies, brownies, doughnuts, croissants, hot and cold breakfast cereals, granola bars, noodle soups, all forms of pasta, and seitan, a vegetarian protein made from wheat. It includes breaded foods and foods made with bread crumbs, such as meatloaf, meatballs, dumplings, tempura, veggie burgers, crab cakes, fish sticks, and deep-fried calamari.

This category also encompasses foods derived from corn—which is a grain, not a vegetable—like cornmeal, corn flour, masa harina, corn syrup, cornstarch, corn oil (and foods fried in corn oil), corn chips, tortillas, tacos, enchiladas, tamales, taquitos, burritos, and fajitas. It includes foods made with these ingredients—such as soups, sauces, gravies, custards, puddings, and pie fillings thickened with cornstarch—and processed foods like cookies, candy, and soda that have been sweetened with corn syrup. Many food additives also come from corn, including citric acid, fructose, food starch, artificial flavoring, natural flavoring, artificial and alternative sweeteners, powdered sugar, glycerin, malt, cellulose gum, xanthan gum, and monosodium glutamate (or MSG), among others. Most processed foods contain some kind of corn.

Whole Grains

This category includes all grains. It's true that whole grains like brown rice have a slight advantage over processed grains like white rice and flour, thanks to very small amounts of protein, fat, and fiber in the intact germ and bran layers. But the bottom line is that they're still mostly starch. The grain category includes all kinds of rice—white, red, brown, black, basmati, jasmine, Forbidden (literally in this case)—as well as wheat berries, buckwheat (kasha), oats and oatmeal, rye, barley, amaranth, millet, quinoa, teff, bulgur, triticale, spelt, corn (maize), and hominy. It also includes any foods made with whole grains, such as rice cakes, popcorn, porridge, grits, polenta, risotto, pilaf, and paella.

Starchy Fruits and Vegetables

Starchy fruits and vegetables include bananas, plantains, all kinds of potatoes (including sweet potatoes), yams, carrots, parsnips, turnips, rutabagas, pumpkins, and winter squashes like acorn, butternut, delicata, and spaghetti squashes. This category also includes food products made from starchy vegetables, like potato starch, potato chips, chips made from other root vegetables, hash browns, Tater Tots, French fries, and sweet-potato fries. It also includes soups, stews, sauces, and gravies that contain these ingredients and processed foods thickened with potato starch. Beets are an exception that will be discussed in chapter 3.

Processed Fruit

Processed fruit includes all fruit that is sweetened or changed in any way from its original whole food form: jelly, jam, dried fruit, canned fruit, fruit concentrates, fruit-juice concentrates, and fruit juice, whether ready-made or fresh squeezed.

Soft Drinks and Milk

Soft drinks include all sweet beverages and sweetened beverages, whether naturally or artificially sweetened, like soda, fruit punch, flavored water, energy drinks, and sports drinks. It also includes iced tea and iced coffee unless they are brewed, unflavored, and unsweetened.

The milk category encompasses all kinds of milk from cows, goats, and sheep: whole, 2 percent, 1 percent, skim, fat-free, and flavored milks like chocolate or strawberry. Milk is a fast carb because it's full of lactose, which is a natural simple sugar. (Fermented dairy products, such as yogurt, are low in lactose because bacteria consume the natural sugars.) Milk also contains natural growth hormones that raise insulin levels through mechanisms independent of its sugar content. One study showed that it doubled fasting insulin levels and the incidence of insulin resistance (Hoppe et al. 2005). Milk can also contain genetically modified growth hormones like recombinant bovine growth hormone (rBGH), also known as recombinant bovine somatotropin (rBST), which is given to cows to increase milk production. These growth hormones also increase the production of insulin-like growth factors that are secreted into milk. They are not destroyed by pasteurization, and inside our bodies, they can act like insulin and promote insulin resistance.

The milk category also includes store-bought nondairy milks: rice milk, soy milk, almond milk, and coconut milk sold as a beverage (it does not include coconut milk intended for cooking that contains only coconut extract and water). These manufactured milks usually contain sweeteners, stabilizers, thickeners, and preservatives. Rice milk also contains inflammatory fats like canola, sunflower, or safflower oil. Homemade nut milks, on the other hand, are acceptable when made with filtered water and raw nuts that have been soaked for twenty-four hours. (Read more about soaking nuts in chapter 8.) Just blend them together, using more water for a milk-like consistency or less water for a cream-like consistency.

The long lists above can be discouraging, but there is some good news. There are plenty of carbohydrates that are safe for people with prediabetes to eat. You'll learn about them in the next section, and chapter 3 will detail the wide variety of other foods that are also good choices. Instead of focusing on what you can't eat, focus on what you can eat. After all, optimism is associated with better physical and psychological well-being and longer life spans.

Slow Carbs

Unlike fast carbs, slow carbs come from fibrous and nonstarchy whole foods, and they have minimal impacts on blood sugar and insulin levels, for they are digested and absorbed slowly. These slow carbs include vegetables like artichokes, asparagus, avocados, bell peppers, broccoli, brussels sprouts, celery, cabbage, cauliflower, collard greens, cucumber, eggplant, endive, kale, leeks, lettuce, mushrooms, mustard greens, okra, onions, peppers, radishes, salad greens, spinach, string beans, Swiss chard, summer squash, tomatoes, and zucchini. They include fermented vegetables (like sauerkraut, pickles, olives, and capers) and sea vegetables (like hijiki, kombu, nori, and wakame). They also include nuts, seeds, and beans.

Inflammation

Our intake of carbohydrates and their effects on insulin levels are important factors in the development of diabetes, but they aren't the only ones. Chronic or long-term inflammation also promotes diabetes, and it can be caused by a number of factors, including free radicals, advanced glycosylation end-products, too much body fat, unhealthy fats in our diet, and toxic chemicals in the environment.

Free Radicals

Free radicals are natural by-products of metabolism, and they're produced when cells burn sugar for energy. Free radicals are unstable atoms or groups of atoms that have lost one or more electrons through a chemical reaction called *oxidation*. (Atoms are the basic building blocks of living organisms, and electrons are the negatively charged particles attached to them.) To get electrons back, free radicals readily react with other molecules. When they steal electrons from other molecules, the other molecules become free radicals themselves, which starts a chain reaction of free-radical production called *oxidative stress*.

When blood sugar levels are low, free radicals are produced in small amounts, and they're normally neutralized by antioxidants. But when levels of blood sugar are high, free radicals are produced in large amounts and they can overwhelm the body's antioxidant reserves. Excessive amounts of free radicals cause inflammation all over the body, wherever blood vessels travel, and on contact, they damage cells, DNA (our genetic material), anti-inflammatory fatty acids, and insulin receptors.

Advanced Glycosylation End-Products

Like free radicals, advanced glycosylation end-products (or AGEs) are a normal part of metabolism, produced when glucose is burned for energy. When blood sugar levels are low, AGEs are formed continuously but at low levels in reversible reactions. When blood sugar levels are high, AGEs are formed faster and the reactions are irreversible, so they accumulate in the body. AGEs interact with receptors on cell surfaces that activate inflammation, and they bind together in a process called *cross-linking*. When cross-linked AGEs build up in tissues, they cause rigidity and interfere with normal structure and function. Cross-linked proteins in cell membranes interfere with the cell's response to insulin. Collagen, a fundamental component of connective tissue, is particularly susceptible to cross-linking. Collagen cross-linking in skin causes it to lose elasticity and take on a prematurely old appearance. Collagen cross-linking in bones, cartilage, and tendons can cause joints to stiffen. In the cornea, lens, and retina of the eye, it can cause browning, opacity, cataract formation, and loss of vision. In nerve endings: peripheral neuropathy. In blood vessels: reduced elasticity, increased pressure, and hypertension. In kidneys: renal failure. In the brain: dementia. AGEs not only cause inflammation and contribute to the development of diabetes, but they also act as key mediators in complications associated with diabetes.

Excess Body Fat

Fat cells, collectively called *adipose tissue*, don't just store fat. They act as an organ and secrete active compounds called *adipokines* into the bloodstream. Adipokines help regulate inflammation as well as appetite, blood pressure, blood clotting, and other important bodily functions. Excess amounts of body fat secrete excess amounts of pro-inflammatory compounds, which increase inflammation throughout the body, promote insulin resistance, and raise the risk for diabetes and other chronic illnesses (Fantuzzi 2005).

Leptin is an adipokine that promotes the development of diabetes through mechanisms independent of inflammation. Under normal circumstances, leptin reduces appetite and makes cells more sensitive to insulin. However, when excess amounts of body fat accumulate and adipose tissue secretes excessive amounts of leptin, cells begin to ignore it. Leptin resistance promotes insulin resistance.

Pro-inflammatory Fats

The fats in our diet can increase or decrease inflammation depending on their chemical structure. All fatty acids are made up of chains of carbon and hydrogen atoms. When every carbon atom in the chain is saturated with hydrogen atoms, it's called a *saturated fat*. Saturated fats are stable, and they have a regular structure that allows them to pack tightly together, so they're solid at room temperature. Coconut oil, butter, and rendered animal fat are all saturated fats. (Foods always contain mixtures of different fatty acids, but for the sake of simplicity, this discussion categorizes these foods based on the types of fat that predominate.)

When carbon atoms in fatty acids are missing hydrogen atoms, they bond with each other instead in a formation called a double bond. These fatty acids are *unsaturated*. If there's just one double bond, it's a *monounsaturated* fatty acid. If there is more than one double bond, it's *polyunsaturated*. Because unsaturated fatty acids are missing hydrogen atoms, they're always ready to react with other molecules in order to gain some, so they're naturally unstable. The more double bonds they have, the more unstable they are. Fatty acids with two double bonds are billions of times more likely to undergo oxidation than fatty acids with only one double bond (Shanahan and Shanahan 2009). Double bonds also change the three-dimensional structure of fats, so they don't pack together as tightly. As a result, they are liquid at room temperature like olive oil, which is monounsaturated, and vegetable oil, which is polyunsaturated.

Excess Omega-6

Our bodies require two types of polyunsaturated fatty acids in particular: omega-3 fats and omega-6 fats. They're called *essential* because we must get them from food. Their name identifies the location of one double bond in their chemical structure. Omega-6 fats are polyunsaturated fatty acids with a double bond before the sixth-to-last carbon in the chain. Omega-3 fats are polyunsaturated fatty acids with a double bond before the third-to-last carbon in the chain.

Omega-3 fats have anti-inflammatory effects in the body. The parent fatty acid of the omega-3 family, alpha-linolenic acid (ALA), is the most abundant fat on the planet. It's concentrated in green leaves because plants use it for photosynthesis. Leafy green vegetables are good sources of omega-3 fats for both humans and animals. Animals that eat a natural diet high in leafy greens (or algae and plankton in the case of fish and seafood) produce meat, eggs, and dairy products that are full of omega-3 fats. Studies confirm that eating grass-fed meat increases levels of omega-3 fatty acids in the body (McAfee et al. 2011).

The parent fatty acid of the omega-6 family is linoleic acid. Plants use it to store energy in their seeds; it converts to the omega-3 alpha-linolenic acid when the seeds germinate and begin photosynthesis. Here, the term *seeds* refers to the reproductive parts of plants, which include grains. Oils extracted from seeds and grains are high in omega-6 fats. Corn oil contains sixty times more omega-6s than omega-3s, and safflower oil contains seventy-seven times more (Sinatra 2007). When we feed grains to animals, their meat, eggs, and milk also contain high amounts of omega-6 fats. A study published in *The New England Journal of Medicine* found that eggs from chickens fed corn contained twenty times more omega-6 fats than omega-3 fats, while eggs from chickens raised on pasture contained roughly equal amounts (Simopoulos 2008).

The actions of omega-6 fats inside our bodies are complex, as they can have both pro-inflammatory and anti-inflammatory effects. The pro-inflammatory activity predominates when we consume them in large amounts, which is almost always the case. Ideally, we should consume a one-to-one ratio of these fats, but experts estimate that most people in the United States eat up to twenty-five times more omega-6s than omega-3s (Allport 2006). The excessive intake of omega-6s creates inflammation throughout the body.

Oxidized Fats

When unsaturated fats are exposed to heat in the presence of oxygen, they can undergo oxidation reactions that create free radicals and trigger inflammation. Oxidized fats include oils that have been extracted with heat, exposed to high temperatures, or stored at room temperature. Even healthy oils like cold-pressed extra-virgin olive oil can quickly become unhealthy and oxidized when stored at room temperature.

Manufactured Fats

Inflammatory fats also include the unnatural ones made by food manufacturers to extend the shelf life of processed products. Chemical reactions like hydrogenation and interesterification change the three-dimensional structure of fatty acids, creating hydrogenated and trans fats that are less susceptible to oxidation and rancidity. But disrupting their chemical structure disrupts the way they work inside our bodies. These unnatural fats cause inflammation and interfere with insulin receptors (Angelieri et al. 2012). Even a small increase in trans-fat intake, only 2 percent, can increase the risk of insulin resistance and diabetes by up to 40 percent (Salmerón et al. 2001).

Saturated fats are neither inflammatory nor unhealthy. In fact, they are some of the healthiest fats because they're stable and not easily oxidized when exposed to heat, which also makes them the best choices for high-temperature cooking. Despite popular myth, saturated fats do not cause heart disease (Siri-Tarino et al. 2010). Like diabetes, cardiovascular disease is largely caused by inflammation. It's initiated by injury to blood vessels, which triggers plaque formation. The same healing mechanism that causes your skin to form a scab when you have a cut causes the lining of your blood vessels to form plaque when it's injured by high levels of blood sugar, toxic chemicals, or inflammatory fats. Studies show that arterial plaque is full of oxidized unsaturated fatty acids, not saturated fats (Felton et al. 1994).

Pro-inflammatory Fats Vs. Anti-Inflammatory Fats

Foods Containing Pro-Inflammatory Fatty Acids	Foods Containing Anti-Inflammatory Fatty Acids
Whole grains	Green leafy vegetables
Processed grains	Wild-caught fish and seafood
Meat, eggs, and dairy products from grain-fed animals	Wild game
Liquid oils extracted using heat, including vegetable, canola, corn, cottonseed, peanut, safflower, soybean, and sunflower oil	Meat, eggs, and dairy products from grass-fed and pasture-raised animals
Trans fats	Rendered fat from wild game and pasture-raised or grass-fed meats
Hydrogenated or partially hydrogenated fats and oils	Butter from grass-fed cows
Interesterified fats and oils	Cold-pressed oils, like extra-virgin olive, walnut, and flaxseed oil, stored in the fridge and not heated above 300°F
Margarine and other butter substitutes	Raw nuts and seeds stored in the fridge or freezer
Liquid oils heated to temperatures above 300°F	Fish oil stored in the fridge (liquids) or freezer (capsules)
Liquid oils stored at room temperature	
Raw nuts and seeds stored at room temperature	
Roasted nuts and seeds	
Fish oil stored at room temperature	
Deep-fried foods	
Processed foods	

Environmental Toxins

Toxic chemicals in the environment promote inflammation through more than one mechanism. They too can generate free radicals and cause oxidative stress. And they activate our immune systems because they're foreign to our bodies. Our immune systems use inflammation to protect us from anything that's not a normal part of our physiology, including pathogenic or disease-causing bacteria, viruses, cancer cells, and environmental toxins. These foreign substances trigger an inflammatory response designed to destroy and remove them from the body. Most environmental toxins are difficult to eradicate, so the body does the next best thing: it removes them from circulation and locks them up inside fat cells to limit their damage. Unfortunately, along the way, environmental toxins can disrupt hormones, injure cells, and make changes to our DNA. The next chapter will explain their harmful effects and how they increase our risk for diabetes.

The Bottom Line

The three most powerful steps you can take to reverse prediabetes are avoiding fast carbs, reducing inflammation, and undergoing detoxification. This chapter covered carbohydrates and inflammation. Chapter 2 focuses on detoxification.

chapter 2

Detox 101

Toxins are chemicals in the environment that are harmful to our health. Most of the time, we can't see or smell or taste them, but toxins are very real and we're exposed to them every day. Our bodies have a hard time excreting these unnatural substances, so they're stored instead, tucked away inside fat cells where they can't do as much damage as they could floating around our bloodstream. Studies show that the amount of toxins in our tissues depends not on how much body fat we have but on how old we are (Hue et al. 2007). The older we get, the more toxins our bodies contain. They start to build up when we're still inside our mothers' wombs and continue to accumulate throughout our lives.

Detoxification is the removal of these harmful chemicals. It can be used annually or semiannually to maintain good health and prevent disease, or it can be used as needed to renew vitality, improve poor health, and reverse chronic conditions like prediabetes. Either way, undertaking a detox program is a big commitment. Detoxification is a complex process, and there are many mechanisms that have to work together to make it successful. This chapter starts with a look at toxins and then explains how the prediabetes detox program works.

How Toxins in Food Relate to Prediabetes

So far, research studies have identified six different toxins that we ingest through food and water that are associated with an increased risk of diabetes, even in small doses that are well below acceptable levels set by the Environmental Protection Agency (EPA) (Lee et al. 2010). These dietary diabetogens include pesticides (Lee et al. 2010), heavy metals (Chen et al. 2009), bisphenol A (Alonso-Magdalena et al. 2010), phthalates (Svensson et al. 2011), dioxins (Wang et al. 2008), and perfluorinated chemicals used to make nonstick materials (Lin et al. 2009). They promote the development of diabetes through at least four different mechanisms: cellular damage, mitochondrial damage, hormone disruption, and epigenetic changes.

Cell Damage

Environmental toxins can damage insulin-producing cells in the pancreas (Ropero et al. 2008). If the pancreas doesn't make enough insulin, blood sugar levels rise, and so does the risk for diabetes.

Mitochondrial Damage

Chemicals in the environment can also damage specific parts of cells called *mitochondria*, organelles that combine sugar and oxygen to generate energy. This damage isn't limited to the pancreas, and it can happen to cells all over the body. Mitochondria consume more than 80 percent of the oxygen we inhale, and they create more than 90 percent of the energy our cells require. Our bodies contain about five hundred trillion mitochondria, and when they don't function properly, neither do the cells or the tissues and organs they make up. Mitochondrial damage has been linked to fatigue, insulin resistance, and diabetes (Wang, Wang, and Wei 2010).

Hormone Disruption

Environmental toxins that disrupt hormones in the body are called *endocrine disruptors*. They mimic the sex hormone estrogen, elevate levels of insulin, and promote insulin resistance (Alonso-Magdalena, Quesada, and Nadal 2011). Because these chemicals also promote fat accumulation and weight gain independent of diet and exercise, sometimes they are also called *obesogens* (Chen, Brown, and Russo 2009).

Epigenetic Changes

Scientists once thought that our genes are set in stone and cannot be altered. But more modern research shows that our genes are dynamic and adaptable, and that such environmental factors as chemical exposure, diet, exercise, and stress have a significant impact on our DNA. These factors cannot alter the sequence of our genetic code, but they can interact with attachments on genes that activate and inactivate them, turning them on and off (Ornish et al. 2008). These are called *epigenetic* changes because they aren't happening to genetic material, but rather above it. Genes can be passed on to future generations with these attachments intact, causing epigenetic changes to be inherited (Godfrey, Inskip, and Hanson 2011). This means that your chemical exposure (as well as your diet and lifestyle) can affect your children and even your children's children. Research studies show that epigenetic changes triggered by chemicals in the environment can increase the risk of diabetes (Godfrey, Inskip, and Hanson 2011).

A Closer Look at Toxins

Here's a closer look at where environmental chemicals are found and how we are exposed to them.

Pesticides

Pesticides are chemicals used to control or eliminate pests, and they come in many forms: herbicides kill weeds, insecticides kill insects, rodenticides kill rodents, and fungicides kill fungus, mildew, and mold. In the United States, more than five billion pounds of pesticides are applied to our crops every year (EPA 2012b). They soak into the soil, where they're taken up into plants through their root systems and distributed throughout, so we can't just wash them off. They make their way into our bodies by three different mechanisms. First, we eat foods that have been treated with pesticides. Second, we feed pesticide-laden foods to the animals we eat. And third, because pesticides don't break down easily, they persist in the environment, polluting waterways and accumulating in the water we drink and the fish and seafood we eat.

Pesticides have a *half-life* of up to fifteen years, which means that it could take up to fifteen years for half the original amount of the substance to break down on its own. But this term can be deceiving: it doesn't mean that the other half will have broken down after another fifteen years has elapsed. If a compound has a half-life of fifteen years, and you start with 100 units, 50 units will remain after fifteen years. After thirty years, 25 units will remain. After forty-five years, 12.5 units will remain. After sixty years, 6.25 units will remain. After seventy-five years, 3.125 units will remain. The substance may undergo exponential decay, but some small amount will always remain.

Heavy Metals

Heavy metals like mercury, cadmium, arsenic, and nickel enter our diet primarily through drinking water, fish and seafood, and fruits and vegetables sprayed with herbicides or grown in contaminated soil. We can also be exposed to heavy metals through cosmetics, perfumes, antiseptics, diaper products, dental amalgams, cigarette smoke, batteries, energy-efficient light bulbs, fabric softeners, paint, floor polish, photography supplies, tattoo ink, and wood preservatives.

Unlike other toxins, heavy metals aren't stored exclusively inside fat cells. They're also stored in bones and organs—primarily the kidneys, liver, intestines, and brain—where their half-lives are measured in decades. In the brain, mercury has a half-life of twenty years, and in the kidneys, cadmium has a half-life of up to thirty-eight years (ATSDR 2008). In the environment, heavy metals persist even longer. In soil, lead has a half-life of fifty-three thousand years (Angima 2010).

Bisphenol A

Bisphenol A (or BPA) is a chemical used to make the epoxy linings inside food and beverage cans. It's also used to make polycarbonate, a hard, clear plastic, and polystyrene. These materials are found in water bottles, baby bottles, plastic wrap, pizza boxes, Styrofoam cups, egg cartons, takeout containers, coolers, dental fillings, plastic water pipes, and other plastic items. BPA leaches from plastics into foods and beverages we consume, especially when the containers are heated or the contents are hot. Because BPA is fat soluble, it's also more likely to leach into foods and drinks that contain fats and oils. This toxic chemical is also used to make recycled paper, carbonless receipts, compact discs, electronics, medical tubing, and eyeglasses. When plastics are discarded, BPA escapes from landfills and enters waterways, contaminating drinking water, fish, and seafood.

In the year 2000, researchers detected BPA in more than 40 percent of the 139 streams they sampled in thirty states across the United States (Kolpin et al. 2002). The Centers for Disease Control found BPA in every single sample from the 2,500 people studied in its most recent National Health and Nutrition Examination Survey (CDC 2013).

BPA doesn't accumulate inside our bodies the way that other toxins do, and studies show that diet can have dramatic effects. As part of a joint study done by Silent Spring Institute and the Breast Cancer Fund, researchers replaced canned, packaged, and prepared foods with fresh foods for five families for three days and tested levels of BPA metabolites in their urine for eight days. This diet change alone caused BPA levels to drop by 66 percent on average and up to 76 percent (Rudel et al. 2011).

Phthalates

Phthalates are chemicals in plastics that make them flexible. In our diet, we're exposed to them primarily through foods and drinks contained in plastic and epoxy-lined cans. Because phthalates aren't tightly bound to plastic polymers, they are highly susceptible to leaching. They're found in food and beverage cans, plastic food and beverage containers, plastic storage containers, plastic wrap, and certain medications. They can also be found in adhesives, shower curtains, tablecloths, medical devices, plastic toys (children's toys and adult sex toys), vinyl flooring, paint, industrial solvents, automotive products, and personal products. Phthalates in cosmetics, nail polish, perfume, and anything with a fragrance are easily absorbed through the skin.

Like BPA, phthalates were found in every single person studied as part of the National Health and Nutrition Examination Survey. Also like BPA, phthalates don't accumulate in the body. The same study that replaced canned and packaged foods with fresh foods also found great reductions in levels of urinary phthalate metabolites, 56 percent on average and up to 96 percent (Rudel et al. 2011).

Dioxins

Dioxins are produced by volcanoes, forest fires, and chemical plants that make bleached paper and other chlorine-containing compounds. They're also produced when plastics are burned. Examples include polychlorinated biphenyls (PCBs), polychlorinated dibenzofurans (PCDFs), and polychlorinated dibenzodioxins (PCDDs). Once these chemicals are released into the environment, they contaminate soils and waterways and accumulate in our food. More than 90 percent of human exposure to dioxins comes from food, according to the World Health Organization (2010). The greatest source for most people is contaminated fish and seafood, and the highest concentrations are found in predators at the top of the food chain like tuna, swordfish, marlin, and shark. Dioxins have a half-life of up to eleven years.

Perfluorinated Chemicals

Perfluorinated chemicals (or PFCs) make materials stain resistant and stick resistant. Several PFCs exist, but the two most common are perfluorooctanoic acid (or PFOA) and perfluorooctane sulfonate (or PFOS). They leach into our food from nonstick cookware and from food packaging like pizza boxes, microwave popcorn bags, and fast food containers. PFCs have "thousands of important manufacturing and industrial applications," according to the EPA, and they're also found in fabric, furniture, carpet, clothing, cleaning products, and personal-care products (EPA 2013). PFCs have a half-life of up to eight and a half years.

What Detox Is

Detoxification is the removal of toxins, and it's something that our bodies do naturally. In fact, your body is doing it right now. Every single second, our cells are generating energy and generating waste products as a normal part of metabolism, and every single second, our bodies are working to eliminate the waste products.

The same mechanisms that help our bodies excrete natural waste products also help excrete unnatural products like toxic compounds from the environment. But in our modern world, where we're continuously exposed to high concentrations of harmful chemicals, it can be difficult to keep up, and toxins can overwhelm our capacity to eliminate them. When there are more toxins coming in than our bodies can excrete, they are stored instead. Most environmental toxins are fat soluble, so they're stored in fat cells, and it can be difficult to get them out, especially when high levels of insulin trap them inside.

There are several things we can do to enhance our body's natural ability to eliminate the toxic chemicals we take in. When we apply these methods for a specified period of time, we can call it a detoxification program. I'll explain the details of the prediabetes detox soon, but first, a basic understanding of our natural detoxification mechanisms is in order.

Detoxification involves several hormones, enzymes, and organs, including the liver, kidneys, gastrointestinal tract, skin, lungs, adipose tissue, and lymphatic system. It happens in three steps: mobilization, detoxification, and elimination.

Mobilization

The extent to which toxins accumulate inside our bodies depends on what we are exposed to and what we eat and drink. When we consume foods and beverages that raise blood sugar and insulin levels, environmental toxins are stored inside adipose cells along with fatty acids, and they remain trapped there as long as insulin levels are high. But when we eat a diet that keeps blood sugar and insulin levels low, our bodies release fatty acids to be burned for energy and, at the same time, toxins are released back into the bloodstream.

The lymphatic system also plays an important role in mobilization. It's a network of vessels, ducts, nodes, and glands that filters body fluids and removes waste products and toxins from cells like an extensive garbage collection system. It returns these compounds, destined for elimination, to the bloodstream. Once toxins are back in the blood, whether they are released from fat cells directly or collected by the lymphatic system, they travel to the liver.

Detoxification

The liver is the largest organ inside the body, and it has many important jobs: changing sugar to fat and fat to sugar; producing bile, a fluid that helps digest fat and releases waste products into the gastrointestinal tract; removing hormones, supplements, and medications from circulation; and detoxifying dangerous chemicals. Your liver lives just beneath the lower portion of your rib cage on the right side, and at any given time about 13 percent of your total blood volume is passing through it. When traveling toxins make their way there, chemical reactions transform them into water-soluble compounds that are easier for the body to eliminate. These chemical reactions are dependent on cofactors like vitamins, minerals, antioxidants, and amino acids. Without enough cofactors, detoxification can be compromised.

There are two main chemical pathways that the liver uses to break down toxins: phase 1 and phase 2. First, phase 1 enzymes transform chemicals in the blood into intermediate products. Sometimes intermediate products are less harmful than the original substances, and other times they are more harmful. Free radicals are a by-product of phase 1, and without adequate antioxidants to neutralize them, they damage DNA, insulin receptors, cells, and anti-inflammatory fats inside the body. The most important antioxidant in phase 1 is glutathione. It's found inside every single cell, but liver cells contain the highest concentrations of it. Besides antioxidants, phase 1 chemical reactions require B vitamins, vitamins C and E, selenium, and magnesium.

The phase 2 detoxification pathway adds a new molecule to the intermediate products from phase 1, changing them into water-soluble compounds. This is critically important, because if phase 2 isn't efficient, intermediate products that are more dangerous than the original substances can wreak havoc inside our bodies. Water-soluble compounds leave the liver through the bloodstream, where they travel to organs of elimination, or through the bile, which is secreted into the intestines and excreted with the stool. In addition to vitamins and minerals, the chemical reactions in phase 2 require amino acids like taurine, glutamine, glycine, and cysteine that come from protein. Taurine also helps improve cells' sensitivity to insulin. A form of cysteine called N-acetylecysteine (NAC) also increases glutathione levels and helps the body excrete methylmercury, the form of mercury found in fish.

The word "detoxification" can be confusing, for it has two meanings. It can refer to this second step involving biochemical pathways in the liver. It can also refer to the general removal of toxins from the body, which involves all three steps. Throughout the rest of this book, unless specified otherwise, "detoxification" or "detox" will refer to the entire process, or all three steps.

Elimination

Once the liver has changed fat-soluble toxins into water-soluble compounds, they are ready to be eliminated from the body, so it's essential that the routes of elimination are all working properly. If they aren't, toxins can be redeposited inside fat cells.

The four organs of elimination are the intestines, kidneys, skin, and lungs.

Intestines

Our intestines excrete toxins with our stool. Because bowel movements are one of the most important ways that your body excretes toxins, they must be regular. If you're not having at least one bowel movement every day, this must be addressed before you begin the detox program (skip ahead to chapter 4 and read the section on treating constipation). Ideally, you should have one bowel movement after each meal you eat. Stools should be brown in color and formed, they should be soft and easy to pass, and they should sink to the bottom of the toilet bowl. Having three bowel movements per day is normal as long as stools aren't watery, explosive, uncomfortable, or accompanied by mucus, blood, or undigested food. If your bowel movements are uncomfortable or abnormal in any way, you should see a naturopathic doctor before you start the detox. If you have acute intestinal inflammation, this too must be addressed before beginning detoxification.

Kidneys

Kidneys excrete toxins through the urine. To ensure that they're efficiently removing toxins processed by the liver, you need to drink plenty of water. If you have kidney disease or if your doctor has told you to limit your intake of fluids for any reason, you should not undergo detoxification. If you have any concerns, your doctor can order simple blood and urine tests to evaluate your kidney function, such as blood urea nitrogen (BUN) and creatinine clearance.

Skin and Lungs

Our bodies eliminate toxins and waste products through the lungs when we exhale and through the skin when we sweat. The skin is the largest organ in the body and has about eighteen square feet of surface area. That's a lot of opportunity for elimination.

Exercise increases circulation throughout the body and promotes the excretion of toxins through both sweat and increased air exchange, so it's an important part of detoxification. Regular physical activity is also essential for improving insulin sensitivity, reversing prediabetes, and maintaining good mental and physical health.

Other ways to increase the elimination of environmental toxins through sweat involve raising your body temperature. Our bodies are always aiming for *homeostasis*, a stable internal environment, and tightly regulate our temperature. Sweat is our built-in cooling system, and when we get too hot, our bodies increase circulation to the skin surface and we release some of the heat through our sweat glands. Saunas are an effective way to induce sweating and eliminate environmental toxins (Dahlgren et al. 2007), but hot baths also work (see chapter 5). Plants called *diaphoretics* also increase sweating. Examples include ginger, cayenne, and cinnamon.

What Detox Is Not

Detox products and protocols are everywhere these days, from raw food and vegan diets to footbaths and body wraps. But detoxification can only happen when the body is burning fat for energy. Unless insulin levels remain low and sugar isn't widely available, the body will always store fat and toxins, never release them. Simply eating raw food, adopting a vegan diet, soaking your feet, or nourishing your skin is not detoxification. These things may be good for us (or not), and they may help minimize our exposure to toxins, but they don't detoxify our bodies.

The low blood sugar and low insulin levels necessary for detoxification can be achieved by eating a diet low in sweets and starches, but most popular "detox" protocols include foods, drinks, and/or supplements that can raise blood sugar levels, like juice, whole grains, starchy fruits and vegetables, and even products containing natural and artificial sweeteners. As a result, elevations in blood sugar and insulin cause toxins to be stored rather than released, and detoxification doesn't happen.

Another popular method of detoxification is calorie restriction or fasting. Both will lower blood sugar and insulin levels, but without adequate protein and the necessary nutrients to drive phase 1 and phase 2 reactions in the liver, detoxification mechanisms are compromised. Toxins that have been released from fat cells can build up to harmful levels in the body. Unsupervised fasting can be dangerous, so never attempt this on your own.

Prediabetes Detox Program Overview

Now it's time to get into the nuts and bolts of the prediabetes detox program. Here you can get a general idea of everything involved. The next three chapters will go into the details of the diet, supplements, and lifestyle factors that will be critical for your success.

Prediabetes Detox Dietary Guidelines

The prediabetes detox diet is designed to lower levels of blood sugar and insulin, burn fat, mobilize and eliminate stored toxins, and reverse prediabetes. There are fourteen dietary guidelines:

1. Avoid fast carbs like sweets, starches, and processed foods.

2. Avoid inflammatory fats.

3. Eat three satisfying meals each day and fast for twelve hours overnight.

4. Consume two tablespoons of ground flaxseeds each day.

5. Eat organic whenever possible.

6. Eat at least two cups of liver-supportive foods every day.

7. Eat fermented foods every day.

8. Dairy products are optional.

9. Choose fish and seafood high in omega-3 fats and low in toxins.

10. Consume only wild, pasture-raised, and grass-fed meat, egg, and dairy products, or none at all.

11. Season food with cinnamon, ginger, cayenne, garlic, onions, fenugreek, cumin, turmeric, black pepper, parsley, cilantro, vinegar, and citrus zest.

12. Avoid foods and beverages in contact with plastic, polystyrene, and nonstick surfaces.

13. Take your weight in pounds and drink half that number in ounces of filtered water every day. (A 150-pound person should drink at least seventy-five ounces of water daily.)

14. Include three or more cups of hot or cold unsweetened tea as part of your daily water intake.

Prediabetes Detox Supplements

You should use certain supplements during detoxification to guarantee that you get the necessary nutrients and cofactors that your liver needs. I recommend a good-quality multivitamin/mineral (MVM) formula, extra vitamin C and magnesium, vitamin D, antioxidant alpha lipoic acid, anti-inflammatory omega-3 fats, probiotics, and a botanical (herbal) supplement to optimize liver function, protect your liver from the dangerous toxins it processes, and improve elimination. You'll take these supplements three times per day with food. (See chapter 4 for a detailed explanation, along with guidelines for selecting high-quality supplements.) You can find recommendations for specific products at www.prediabetesdetox.com.

Prediabetes Detox Lifestyle

The prediabetes detox lifestyle has five basic guidelines:

1.   Stop smoking.

2.   Exercise for five hours each week.

3.   Manage stress effectively.

4.   Get at least nine hours of sleep each night.

5.   Take saunas regularly, or take warm Epsom salt baths.

Many of these lifestyle components will fit into your regular routine. Others will take more time, and you'll need to find a way to work them into your daily schedule. Don't think of new activities as additional burdens. Think of them as permanent changes. Healthy meals, regular physical activity, and adequate sleep support detoxification and play an important role in reversing prediabetes as well as other chronic illnesses. You'll want to make them a part of your life forever.

Duration

You should follow the prediabetes detox program for at least two weeks and until your blood sugar levels have normalized. You should be testing your fasting blood sugar level every morning when you wake up, before you have anything to eat or drink. After two weeks, if your fasting blood sugar level is not yet consistently below eighty-one milligrams per deciliter, continue the detox program until it is or for six more weeks (eight weeks total), whichever comes first. How long it takes for you to achieve normal blood sugar levels will depend on the severity of your blood sugar imbalance, your commitment to following the program, and your body's natural capacity for healing.

What to Expect

When your body starts to detoxify, you may feel worse before you feel better. It happens because chemicals that have been tucked away are suddenly released back into your bloodstream and circulate throughout your entire body. You may feel better right away, but it's not uncommon to experience fatigue, headaches, nausea, food cravings, mood swings, irritability, skin rashes, flu-like symptoms, lethargy, brain fog, and general dis-ease. Many of these symptoms are usually short lived, lasting for just two or three days, until your liver function catches up to its new workload and your body begins to clear toxins more efficiently. After that, most people start to feel better than they have in a long time. My patients frequently tell me that they had forgotten how good feeling good feels, because they had gotten so used to feeling bad. Detoxification reminded them.

Some symptoms take longer to resolve. Food cravings related to high levels of blood sugar and insulin should go away when blood sugar and insulin levels normalize, and symptoms of caffeine withdrawal can persist for up to a week, depending on how much you're used to consuming. If you drink more than one cup of coffee per day, consider cutting back before you begin the detox program.

During detoxification, it's also possible to experience an aggravation of physical, mental, or emotional conditions that you already have, like eczema or depression. Recognize that detox is an opportunity to release toxic emotions as well as physical toxins.

On a positive note, for people who are overweight, weight loss is usually a side effect of detoxification. As you eliminate fast carbs from your diet and your blood sugar levels drop, your body will automatically burn fat for energy. Losing stores of fat results in a leaner body and weight loss for most people. But if you don't lose weight, don't worry. It isn't a prerequisite for reversing prediabetes. Studies show that an intensive program of diet and exercise that lowers insulin levels can reverse prediabetes even when people don't lose weight (Barnard et al. 1992).

If you experience any symptoms that do not resolve within eight weeks, you should see a physician, for you may have a deeper imbalance that must be addressed. I highly recommend looking for a licensed naturopathic doctor if you don't have one already. See www. prediabetesdetox.com for more information about naturopathic doctors and how to find one in your area.

Precautions

The prediabetes detox program is safe for most people, but some should not participate, and others should seek the advice of their doctor before they begin. If you are pregnant or breastfeeding, you should not undergo detoxification, for environmental toxins are especially harmful to babies. In pregnant women, environmental toxins can be transferred to fetuses, and in lactating women, toxins can be eliminated through breast milk. You should not undergo detox if you have kidney disease, liver disease, cardiac arrhythmia, unexplained abdominal pain, or acute inflammation of any part of the gastrointestinal tract, including the gallbladder, pancreas, and intestines. If you've had recent surgery or chemotherapy treatments, you should wait until you're fully recovered and seek approval from your naturopathic doctor before starting detoxification. Again, if you are not having regular bowel movements (at least one per day), resolve this issue before starting detoxification (see chapter 4).

If you have serious health problems or take prescription medications, you should talk to your doctor before you begin detoxification. Increasing liver function can alter the metabolism of certain drugs, so your doctor may need to adjust your dosage. If you haven't been exercising, you should see your doctor and get permission to exercise before you begin detoxification. If your doctor isn't trained in detoxification, I highly recommend looking for a licensed naturopathic doctor.

Detox Tools

Besides groceries and supplements, you'll need these tools for the prediabetes detox program:

- Blood sugar monitor
- Water filter
- Grinder for flaxseeds (either electric or mortar and pestle)
- Access to a sauna or bathtub
- Journal
- Calendar

The journal is optional, but I highly recommend it. Keeping a record of your activities, symptoms, and feelings can provide useful feedback, foster a sense of accountability, and motivate you to achieve your goals. You'll need a calendar to appoint a start date for the detox program, schedule activities like exercise, and set aside time to shop for food, prepare healthy meals, and get plenty of sleep. The first three days of the detox program are usually the most difficult, so if you can, plan them to coincide with the weekend or whenever you have fewer work and social responsibilities. If possible, avoid detox when under the weather or during periods of travel, sudden grief, or other acute physical and emotional upsets. Also realize that the time may never be absolutely perfect, so pick a start date in the near future and stick to it.

It's also helpful to have basic kitchen equipment for preparing healthy meals and at least one good cookbook. If you're new to cooking, you can find a list of kitchen staples, recommended cookbooks, and healthy recipes at www.prediabetesdetox.com.

Daily Detox Checklist

To make this program easy to follow, you can download a daily detox checklist from www.prediabetesdetox.com. The seven-day checklist will help you keep track of your morning fasting glucose levels and allow you to check off your daily dietary goals, the supplements you're taking, and the lifestyle activities that are part of the program. You can make notes and add items of your own if you want to personalize the program to help you meet specific goals. Print out as many copies as you need.

chapter 3
Prediabetes Detox Diet

It's important to make a firm commitment to the basic dietary guidelines during the prediabetes detox. If you don't follow the guidelines closely, your blood sugar and insulin levels can remain elevated, which means that your body won't be able to detoxify itself, and prediabetes will continue to progress. Think of the prediabetes detox as a good opportunity to make much-needed changes in both diet and lifestyle. The detoxification program may only last for a couple of weeks, but afterward, many of these principles and practices should become part of your regular routine to permanently reverse prediabetes and reduce your risk of chronic illness.

This chapter discusses the fourteen guidelines of the prediabetes detox diet in detail. I'll also explain how the prediabetes detox diet can be adapted for vegetarians and vegans, and at the end of the chapter you'll find some simple but specific lists of which foods to eat and which ones to avoid. If you need ideas for turning the foods you can eat into healthy and satisfying meals, visit www.prediabetesdetox.com for sample menus. There you'll find three sets of weeklong menus: one for omnivores, one for people following a dairy-free diet, and another for vegetarians.

1. Avoid Sweets, Starches, and Processed Foods

Eating a diet low in fast carbohydrates is the most powerful step you can take to detox successfully and reverse prediabetes permanently. In fact, you can't accomplish these things without it. Here's a quick reminder of the fast carbs you should avoid during detoxification:

- All sweeteners, whether natural or artificial, and sweetened foods
- All grains, including rice, oatmeal, and corn
- Foods made with flour, including bread, pastries, crackers, breakfast cereals, and pasta
- Starchy fruits and vegetables like bananas, potatoes, carrots, and winter squashes
- Processed fruit like jam, jelly, dried fruit, and fruit juice
- Soft drinks, including soda, flavored water, energy drinks, and sports drinks
- Milk
- Alcohol, including beer and wine

See chapter 1 for more detailed lists of these foods.

2. Avoid Inflammatory Fats

Here's a reminder of what you want to avoid:

- Vegetable oil, canola oil, corn oil, cottonseed oil, peanut oil, safflower oil, soybean oil, sunflower oil, and all colorless, flavorless oils
- Liquid oils heated to temperatures above 300°F
- Deep-fried foods

- Processed and manufactured foods, especially those containing liquid oils, trans fats, and hydrogenated, partially hydrogenated, or interesterified oils

- Fake butter products like margarine and vegetable oil spreads and sprays

- Roasted and toasted nuts and seeds in any form

- Grains, flours, and foods made from flour

- Grain-fed animal products like meat, eggs, and dairy products

You can review the more detailed lists of inflammatory fats in chapter 1.

3. Eat Regular Meals and Fast Overnight

Eating three regular meals each day and fasting for twelve hours overnight maximizes detoxification and keeps blood sugar and insulin levels low for extended periods of time. A study from Harvard University that followed almost thirty thousand people for sixteen years found that people who ate three regular meals each day and did not snack had a significantly lower risk of developing diabetes than those who skipped breakfast and those who ate more frequently, regardless of body mass index and food quality (Mekary et al. 2012).

If you're used to eating a lot of fast carbs, your body is used to burning sugar for fuel, and it may take some time for your body to adjust to burning fat for fuel instead. During this transition, you may experience symptoms of hypoglycemia, like intense hunger, sweating, dizziness, nervousness, weakness, and confusion. If you experience any of these symptoms, have a small snack that contains slow carbs, healthy fat, and protein. Here are some suggestions:

- Celery sticks with almond butter

- Cucumber rounds with hummus

- Fresh berries and raw nuts

- A pickle and a piece of cheese or a hard-boiled egg
- Soup
- Leftovers
- Dark Chocolate Coconut Clusters (see recipe in chapter 8)

Once your body begins to better regulate levels of blood sugar and insulin, hunger and food cravings will resolve, and snacking shouldn't be an issue, because you won't feel hungry. If you do, it's a sign that your last meal didn't contain adequate amounts of protein, healthy fat, and/or fiber. All three of these macronutrients slow down the digestion and absorption of glucose, which minimizes elevations in blood sugar and insulin levels, reduces food cravings, keeps you satiated between meals, and sustains your energy levels throughout the day. If you're so hungry between meals that you can't wait for the next one, have a small snack like the ones listed above and adjust your next meal accordingly.

Fiber Helps Reverse Prediabetes

A study published in the *New England Journal of Medicine* compared the effects of different amounts of dietary fiber on people with type 2 diabetes (Chandalia et al. 2000). For six weeks, one group consumed a moderate fiber diet (twenty-four grams per day) as recommended by the American Diabetes Association, while the other group ate a high-fiber diet of fifty grams per day. At the end of the trial, researchers concluded that compared to the ADA diet, the high-fiber diet resulted in significantly lower levels of fasting glucose and insulin.

So how much should you eat? Despite what popular diet myths may lead you to believe, there's no magic formula for food intake. Counting calories doesn't work, because it's the quality of foods that matter, not the quantity. (For example, five hundred calories of cookies is not equivalent to five hundred calories of broccoli.) Instead, start with an average dinner plate ten inches in diameter. One-quarter of the plate, a portion roughly equal to the size of your palm, should be protein: meat, fish, eggs, tempeh, or beans. Half of the plate should be green vegetables. Vegetables are good sources of fiber, vitamins, minerals, and antioxidants, and green varieties are also particularly rich in chlorophyll, a compound that reduces the absorption of environmental chemicals and facilitates their removal from the body (Morita, Matsueda, and Iida 1999). The remaining quarter of the plate should contain one or more of the following: more vegetables, raw nuts or seeds, beans (if they weren't your protein source), organic dairy products (if you eat dairy), or fruit (citrus or berries). Somewhere on the plate should be at least one source, and ideally several sources, of healthy fat.

Healthy Fats

Healthy fats come from a variety of sources:

- Cold-pressed oils: extra-virgin olive, coconut, walnut, and flaxseed
- Olives
- Avocados
- Raw nuts and seeds, especially almonds, which have been found to lower levels of blood sugar and hemoglobin A1C (Cohen and Johnston 2011), and those highest in omega-3 fats, including walnuts (which are also a good source of glutathione), macadamia nuts, ground flax-seeds, and chia seeds
- Unsweetened raw nut butter
- Unsweetened coconut, fresh or dried
- Unsweetened coconut milk
- Nontoxic fish and seafood
- Wild game and pasture-raised or grass-fed eggs, meat, dairy products, including butter and ghee, and rendered animal fat
- Cocoa butter in dark chocolate (85 percent dark, limited to one ounce per day)

Always buy cold-pressed liquid oils, store them in the fridge, and never heat them above 300°F. Because olive oil solidifies in the fridge, if you use it frequently, keep a small amount in an opaque or dark glass bottle at room temperature and refill it as needed.

If you prefer the flavor of roasted nuts and seeds, toast them yourself in a dry skillet over low heat until fragrant and lightly browned and eat them immediately. Don't toast them in advance to store for future use.

Unscientific as it may sound, you'll find what's right for you through trial and error. Eat slowly, take time to chew your food well, and stop when you're no longer hungry. You should never feel too full after you eat. Studies show that the faster you eat, the more likely you are to develop diabetes (Radzevičienė and Ostrauskas 2012), and that chewing food at least thirty times before swallowing has a positive influence on key mediators that help regulate appetite, food intake, blood sugar, and body weight (Saito, Hattori, and Eto 2011). You should chew your food so thoroughly that it's nearly liquid before you swallow it. If you're used to rushing through meals, slow down and count your chews.

To keep blood sugar and insulin levels low for an extended period of time, meals should be spaced at least five or six hours apart, and there should be a twelve-hour period of fasting between dinner and breakfast. Fasting is an effective method for mobilizing stored toxins, but it can be dangerous when used alone (see chapter 2). A twelve-hour overnight fast is a safe and effective way to incorporate fasting into a comprehensive detox program. You shouldn't be hungry overnight, because when you're sleeping, high levels of the hormone melatonin naturally suppress your appetite. Nighttime hunger may be a symptom of high insulin levels, or a sign that you need to make changes to your sleeping environment (see chapter 5).

4. Consume Two Tablespoons of Ground Flaxseeds Daily

Ground flaxseeds are an excellent tool for both detoxification and reversing prediabetes. They help eliminate toxins from the body, reduce the absorption of carbohydrates, support the growth of healthy bacteria, and improve insulin sensitivity and blood sugar control (Mani et al. 2011). They're also very high in anti-inflammatory omega-3 fatty acids. Whole flaxseeds usually pass through our digestive tract intact, so to access all of the beneficial compounds inside, you'll have to grind them before you eat them. It's easiest to do with a clean electric coffee or spice grinder (don't use a grinder you use for coffee beans to grind flaxseeds unless it can be thoroughly washed), but you can also use a mortar and pestle if you like. Grind them fresh each day, or you can grind a cup or so at a time as needed and keep them in an airtight glass jar in the fridge to prevent oxidation of their fragile fatty acids. Preground flaxseeds are available in health-food stores, but because they are exposed to heat and light during processing and transport, you should buy them whole and grind them yourself. It's not only better for you, but it's also much less expensive.

Ground flaxseeds have a coarse texture and a nutty flavor. They absorb a lot of moisture in your digestive tract, so you should consume them with at least eight ounces of water to prevent constipation. I find it easiest to add them to a smoothie (see recipe in chapter 8), but you can also stir them into yogurt or sprinkle them over soups and salads. Once they come into contact with moisture, they gradually thicken and develop a mucilaginous quality, so you should consume them right away.

Although ground flaxseeds benefit most people, a small percentage may develop gas, bloating, or loose stools. Sometimes these symptoms are temporary and resolve once your digestive system becomes accustomed to the extra fiber. If you experience any gastrointestinal discomfort that is severe or does not resolve within three or four days, discontinue the ground flaxseeds and replace them with one tablespoon of psyllium seed husk. The fiber in psyllium has also been shown to lower high levels of blood sugar and insulin (Pastors et al. 1991). Look for a pure product that contains only powdered psyllium husk, and avoid products like Metamucil that contain sweeteners, artificial flavors, and food coloring. As with ground flaxseeds, you can add psyllium husk powder to a smoothie or stir it into eight ounces of water. Drink it immediately and follow it with two additional cups of water because psyllium will absorb a lot of water in your intestines.

Note: If you have bowel obstruction, diverticulitis, or other acute intestinal inflammation, you should not consume flaxseeds or psyllium seeds, and you should not undergo detoxification until these conditions have been resolved.

5. Eat Organic Whenever Possible

Organic foods are produced without pesticides, antibiotics, hormones, synthetic fertilizer, genetically engineered ingredients, or irradiation. As mentioned previously, pesticides and added hormones have been linked to insulin resistance and an increased risk of diabetes. Genetically modified foods carry these same risks.

When we eat genetically modified foods, the modified genes they contain become incorporated into the bacterial cells in our intestines and continue to function, producing genetically modified proteins (including herbicides) long after the original food has passed through our digestive tracts and left our bodies (Netherwood et al. 2004). Genetically modified foods have been linked to changes in fat and carbohydrate metabolism, pancreas and liver problems, disruptions in gut bacteria, and altered expression of genes that control the regulation of insulin (Dean and Armstrong 2009). These foods may be genetically modified:

- Sugar

- Corn and all products made from corn

- Soy and all products made from soybeans

- Canola oil

- Cottonseed oil

- Hawaiian papaya

- Zucchini

- Yellow squash

- Meat, eggs, and dairy products from grain-fed animals

So far, genetically modified foods are not labeled in the United States, and most people eat them every day. Experts estimate that 70 percent of our processed foods contain genetically engineered ingredients and, according to the US Department of Agriculture (USDA), 85 percent of our corn, 90 percent of our canola oil, 91 percent of our soybeans, and 88 percent of our cotton (added to foods as cottonseed oil) is genetically modified (CFS 2013). The only way to avoid genetically modified foods is to eat organic. If you can't eat organic, avoid the foods listed above all together. Some of these foods you'll want to avoid whether or not they are organic; they include sugar, corn, canola oil, cottonseed oil, papaya, and products from grain-fed animals.

To minimize your exposure to pesticides, take some help from the Environmental Working Group (EWG), a nonprofit organization that researches health and the environment. EWG analyzed more than sixty thousand samples of forty-five popular fruits and vegetables that were tested for contamination by the USDA and the Food and Drug Administration (FDA) the way they're usually eaten (washed or peeled) (EWG 2013). Researchers found that certain nonorganic fruits and vegetables contained significantly higher levels of pesticides than others. They named the least contaminated ones the Clean Fifteen and the most contaminated ones the Dirty Dozen Plus, which includes the twelve fruits and vegetables with the highest concentrations of pesticides and two others that were commonly contaminated with highly toxic organophosphate insecticides.

The Dirty Dozen Plus most contaminated fruits and vegetables appear here in descending order (apples are the most toxic):

1. Apples

2. Strawberries

3. Grapes

4. Celery

5. Peaches

6. Spinach

7. Sweet bell peppers

8. Nectarines (imported)

9. Cucumbers

10. Potatoes

11. Cherry tomatoes

12. Chili peppers

13. Leafy greens, including kale and collard greens

14. Summer squash

Avoid the foods listed in the Dirty Dozen Plus unless they are organic.

The Clean Fifteen, the least contaminated fruits and vegetables, appear here in ascending order, with corn the least toxic:

1. Corn

2. Onions

3. Pineapples

4. Avocados

5. Cabbage

6. Frozen sweet peas

7. Papayas

8. Mangoes

9. Asparagus

10. Eggplant

11. Kiwi

12. Grapefruit

13. Cantaloupe

14. Sweet potatoes

15. Mushrooms

When you can't eat organic, replace the Dirty Dozen Plus with the Clean Fifteen fruits and vegetables. Some of them aren't allowed during detox, like corn, mangoes, and melons, but it's good to be aware of the full list, for you may be introducing some of these foods after you finish the detox program. These lists are updated annually. You can always find the link to the most current information at www.prediabetesdetox.com.

6. Eat Two Cups of Liver-Supportive Foods Daily

It's important to eat at least two cups of liver-supportive foods every day during detoxification. Cruciferous vegetables, which belong to the Brassicaceae family, are a rich source of sulfur-containing compounds like isothiocyanates and indoles that boost glutathione levels (Lii et al. 2010) and stimulate phase 1 and phase 2 detoxification pathways in the liver (Fowke et al. 2006). They include:

- Arugula

- Bok choy

- Broccoli

- Brussels sprouts

- Cabbage

- Cauliflower

- Collard greens

- Kale

- Kohlrabi

- Mustard greens

- Radishes

- Swiss chard

- Watercress

These foods also support detoxification:

- Beets

- Dandelion greens

- Artichokes

- Berries, especially blackberries

Beets (Nick 2002) and artichokes (Liska and Bland 2002) contain compounds that reduce inflammation, support detoxification pathways, and promote healthy liver function. Artichokes also act as antioxidants and protect the liver from toxic compounds (Liska and Bland 2002). All berries have antioxidant and anti-inflammatory activity in the body, but blackberries have also been shown to reverse pesticide-inflicted damage (Serraino et al. 2003). Because beets are a root vegetable, their intake should be limited to one half-cup serving no more than two times per day.

7. Eat Some Fermented Foods Every Day

Our bodies are covered with microbes, inside and out. They even outnumber us. The average human body contains ten times more microbial cells than human cells (O'Hara and Shanahan 2006). The friendly bacteria inside our digestive tracts help break down toxins, including pesticides (Cho et al. 2009) and phthalates (Yuan 2002). They help regulate insulin sensitivity (Vrieze et al. 2012), reduce inflammation (Isolauri 2001), strengthen our immune systems (O'Hara and Shanahan 2006), prevent the growth of disease-causing bacteria (Isolauri 2001), secrete hormones that help move food through the gastrointestinal tract (O'Hara and Shanahan 2006), and manufacture nutrients. Friendly bacteria also modulate the expression of genes that influence metabolism and fat deposition, and they even affect the development and function of structural components of the digestive tract, including muscles, nerves, blood vessels, and immune cells (O'Hara and Shanahan 2006).

When you have too many of the bad microbes or not enough of the good ones, an imbalance known as *dysbiosis* develops, and your health suffers. Studies show that dysbiosis is common in people with diabetes (Qin et al. 2012).

Eating these lacto-fermented and cultured foods helps promote the growth of beneficial microorganisms called *probiotics*:

- Yogurt

- Kefir

- Cultured butter (butter made from fermented milk)

- Cheese

- Vinegar

- Pickles, capers, and olives

- Sauerkraut

- Kimchi (fermented vegetables)

- Umeboshi (fermented plums, whole or ground into a paste)

- Tempeh

- Miso (a savory paste made from fermented soybeans and used to make soup)

- Tamari (soy sauce made from fermented soybeans)

- Fish sauce

- Cacao nibs

Like tamari, shoyu is a fermented soy sauce, but unlike tamari, it's made with wheat, so it should be avoided. Wine and kombucha, a sugar-sweetened black tea, are also fermented foods, but you shouldn't drink them during detox. It's okay to use small amounts of dry wine in cooking, but choose a wine that is good enough to drink (avoid cooking wines). During the prediabetes detox, you should eat at least one non-pasteurized lacto-fermented or "live culture" food from the preceding list every day. It's also important to include in your diet *prebiotics*, specific kinds of fiber that stimulate the growth of probiotics. Prebiotics are found in ground flaxseeds, artichokes, asparagus, onions, garlic, and beans.

8. Dairy Products Are Optional

Many people do not tolerate dairy foods well. Cow's milk is one of the eight most common food allergens, along with gluten (a protein found in certain grains, including wheat, barley, rye, bulgur, kamut, spelt, and contaminated oats), eggs, peanuts, tree nuts, fish, shellfish, and soy. According to the United States Food and Drug Administration, these foods are responsible for 90 percent of allergic reactions to foods (USFDA 2012). While some individuals have true food allergies, others have food sensitivities or intolerances. Food allergies are hypersensitive immune reactions to specific foods that occur when the body mistakes substances for dangerous or disease-causing compounds. Food sensitivities and intolerances are adverse reactions that do not involve the immune system. Food sensitivities are nonspecific reactions, and food intolerances refer to a problem with the way that the body processes certain foods or components in foods. For example, people who are lactose intolerant can't digest lactose (milk sugar) because they don't make enough lactase, the enzyme needed to break it down.

If you have an allergy, sensitivity, or intolerance to milk, dairy products, or any other foods, no matter how mild, you should avoid them during detoxification. If you aren't sure, err on the side of caution and avoid them anyway. Eliminating certain foods from your diet and then reintroducing them systematically is a very good way to determine whether or not you have food sensitivities or intolerances. However, if you suspect that you have an allergy to certain foods that could possibly result in *anaphylactic shock* (a sudden and severe life-threatening reaction that involves difficulty breathing or sudden drops in blood pressure), only eat these foods under medical supervision.

To test for a dairy sensitivity or intolerance during the detoxification program, avoid it completely for at least fourteen days but ideally for four to six weeks, then reintroduce it according to the guidelines in chapter 7. The same method can be used to test for other suspected food sensitivities and intolerances.

If you are not sensitive to dairy products, some of them are allowed.

You can have plain whole-milk yogurt, aged and ripened cheeses, butter, and cream, as they are low in natural sugars and high in protein and healthy fat. Commercial yogurts contain fewer beneficial bacteria than homemade yogurt contains, so if you can make your own, do. If you're not a fan of plain yogurt, you can mix it with citrus zest and/or fresh or thawed frozen berries. Traditional versions of kefir, buttermilk, sour cream, cream cheese, and cottage cheese would also qualify, but commercial varieties are usually made from low-fat or nonfat milk and contain additives like modified food starch or cornstarch, stabilizers like carrageenan or guar gum, and sometimes even sweeteners, colors, flavoring, and preservatives. These products are not excluded, but unless you make them yourself, it may be impossible for you to find versions that meet the criteria for dairy.

During detoxification, dairy products must:

- Be made from whole milk (avoid all fat-free and low-fat dairy products)

- Come from pasture-raised or grass-fed cows never exposed to pesticides, antibiotics, hormones, or grain-based feed

- Be free of additives, including emulsifiers, stabilizers, sweeteners, flavoring, coloring, and preservatives

9. Choose Fish and Seafood That Are Low in Toxins

Studies show that eating fish and seafood regularly can reduce your risk of developing diabetes (Villegas et al. 2011). They are a good source of the amino acids needed for phase 2 detoxification (Dannenberg and Yang 1992) and omega-3 fats that reduce inflammation, improve blood sugar metabolism, increase insulin sensitivity (Flachs et al. 2009), and protect the brain from pesticide-induced damage (Crinnion 2000). Two of these essential fatty acids, docosahexaenoic acid (DHA) and eicosapentaenoic acid (EPA), are only found in substantial amounts in fish and marine animals. Technically, they're also found in algae—which is why the fish that eat them are such good sources—but the edible varieties don't contain enough DHA and EPA to meet human needs. (Nori and hijiki contain such miniscule amounts that their nutrition labels report zero grams of fat.) The liver can convert other omega-3s to DHA and EPA, but some people don't make enough of the enzyme necessary for the reaction, and according to research studies, the process is "unreliable" and "severely restricted" (Gerster 1998, 159). So we have to get these essential fats from fish and seafood.

Unfortunately, as our oceans and waterways become more polluted, so do our fish and seafood. Environmental toxins like pesticides, dioxins, and heavy metals that don't break down easily persist in the environment for long periods of time and accumulate in animals. Large predatory fish naturally accumulate the most of these toxins while smaller species living lower on the food chain usually accumulate the least.

As global demand for fish and seafood continues to grow, wild fisheries are becoming depleted and fishing practices are damaging the environment. *Aquaculture*, or fish farming, has helped take pressure off wild fisheries, but like confined animal-feeding operations on land, excessive amounts of waste are generated and animals are treated with chemical agents to increase growth and control infections. Surrounding waters become polluted with fish feces, food waste, antibiotics, insecticides, and pesticides. This promotes the growth of oxygen-depleting microorganisms, upsets ecosystems, and threatens wild populations. Farm-raised fish contain significantly higher levels of toxic chemicals, and because they don't eat their natural diet, they don't contain the same healthy omega-3 fats found in wild species.

To find fish that are high in omega-3 fats, low in toxic chemicals, and sustainably harvested, take some help from the experts. The Environmental Defense Fund offers a free online Seafood Selector that rates fish and seafood based on their environmental impact, gives details on health advisories regarding unsafe levels of toxins, and even notes which species are especially good sources of omega-3s. The Seafood Watch Program from the Monterey Bay Aquarium has a similar database as well as region-specific pocket guides and mobile applications (you can find both links at www .prediabetesdetox.com).

At the time of this writing, the best choices in fish and seafood are:

- Wild salmon from Alaska

- Sablefish (black cod) from the United States or Canada

- Herring

- Atlantic mackerel from Canada

- Pacific sardines from the United States

- Pacific halibut from Alaska or Canada

- Anchovies

- Rainbow trout

- Arctic char

- Oysters

Most rainbow trout, Arctic char, and oysters available for purchase in the United States are farm raised, but unlike other farm-raised species, they are high in omega-3 fats, and the aquaculture systems have a low impact on the environment, good control of waste products, and minimal rates of escape into the wild (Weinstein 2006).

Some other fish and seafood have fewer omega-3 fats, but they are low in toxins, can be sustainably harvested, and contain healthy amounts of amino acids needed for phase 2 detox. They're the next best thing:

- Clams

- Mussels

- Scallops

- Dungeness crab (avoid blue crab)

- Wild-caught spiny lobster

- Squid

- Haddock

- Atlantic pollock

- Wild-caught pink shrimp

- Wild-caught spot prawns

Many of these options are also inexpensive and easy to cook.

Always avoid species that contain dangerous levels of environmental contaminants. The worst choices are:

- Farm-raised salmon

- Wild salmon from Washington, Oregon, and California

- King mackerel

- White, albacore, or bluefin tuna

- Bluefish

- Blue crab

- Chilean sea bass

- Tilapia

- Flounder

- Marlin

- Orange roughy

- Rockfish

- Shark

- Snapper

- Sturgeon

- Swordfish

- Large halibut

- Tilefish

- Walleye

- Yellow perch

- Lingcod

- Opah

10. Eat Pasture-Raised, Grass-Fed Meat, Eggs, and Dairy

When it comes to the animals in our diet, it's their diet that matters most. Animals raised in confined animal-feeding operations (CAFOs) eat grains instead of grass, which makes their meat, eggs, and dairy products high in pro-inflammatory omega-6 fats. Grain-based animal feeds also contain additives like artificial flavors, pesticides, and even industrial waste, as well as pharmaceutical drugs, including tranquilizers, cardiac stimulants, anti-inflammatory medications, antibiotics, antiparasitic drugs, growth-promoting hormones, and sex hormones (Epstein 1990). We may not be able to taste pesticides, hormones, antibiotics, or heavy metals, but studies confirm that they end up in meat on supermarket shelves (USDA 2010).

When we eat meat, eggs, and dairy products from grain-fed animals, the chemicals in their bodies end up in our bodies, and even the USDA (2010, 28) warns that these "residues may produce toxic or allergic reactions" in humans. Pesticides, hormones, and heavy metals increase the risk for diabetes directly, and antibiotics increase the risk indirectly by reducing the populations of beneficial bacteria inside the digestive tract.

Compared to meat from CAFOs, grass-fed meat is a much healthier choice. It contains more glutathione, vitamin E, carotenoids (precursors to vitamin A), and conjugated linoleic acid, a fatty acid found to reduce the number of fat cells (Fischer-Posovszky et al. 2007) and cut the risk of diabetes (Daley et al. 2010). While meat from animals raised in CAFOs contains unnaturally high amounts of fat, pasture-raised and grass-fed animals contain a natural fatty acid profile similar to what we see in wild animals: more anti-inflammatory omega-3 fats, fewer pro-inflammatory omega-6 fats, and less total fat (Daley et al. 2010). Our bodies certainly need fat, but it's important not to overconsume fat from animal sources. Like humans, animals are high on the food chain, and even pasture-raised animals can accumulate toxins through environmental pollution. Make plant foods the foundation of your diet and use meat as more of a condiment, to add protein, healthy fat, flavor, and texture to meals.

During the prediabetes detox diet, wild game and pasture-raised or grass-fed meats and animal products are allowed. You'll find a comprehensive list at the end of this chapter.

Mystery Meats

When it comes to buying meat, labels can be difficult to interpret and even misleading. Here's what you need to know:

Grass-fed meat means exactly that: meat from animals that ate grass. It applies to ruminant animals like cows, buffalo, goats, and sheep. Certification by the American Grassfed Association guarantees that the animals were raised only on mother's milk and forage, they were neither fed grains nor administered antibiotics or hormones, and they were given continuous access to pasture.

Pastured or *pasture-raised* meats come from animals that foraged for their food but ate more than grass and green plants. This term applies to omnivores like chickens and pigs. It doesn't have a legal definition, so it is more description than label. You may see this term used at the farmers' market, where people sell the meat they raised, and they're usually happy to tell you how they did it.

The next best thing to eating grass-fed or pasture-raised animal products is eating those high in *omega-3* fats. Studies show that giving animals fish extracts, algae extracts, or flaxseeds significantly enriches the concentration of DHA in their meat and eggs. A French study found increases that were twofold in beef, sixfold in eggs, sevenfold in chicken, and twentyfold in salmon (Bourre 2005).

Labels that read *vegetarian-fed* assure consumers that the animals were not fed other animals. Vegetarian-fed meats and eggs come from grain-fed animals. (If they'd had the chance to eat bugs and worms, they wouldn't be vegetarians.) Remember that certain animals, like chickens and pigs, are omnivores, and their natural diets are not vegetarian.

Labels that say *free range* or *free roaming* only mean that animals had access to the outdoors. It doesn't mean that they were frolicking on a farm, foraging for their food, or that they ever ate a green leafy plant. These animals usually eat grain.

Grain-finished meat comes from animals raised on grass and fattened with grain.

The *organic* label means that the meat was produced without exposure to pesticides, antibiotics, hormones, synthetic fertilizer, genetically engineered ingredients, or irradiation. Organic meats and eggs come from animals fed organic grains, which are better than pesticide-treated grains, but ultimately, they're still grains. Organic meat is a step up from nonorganic meat, but it's not as good as grass-fed or pasture-raised meat.

Note that the label *natural* gives no information about the diet of the animal at all. It just means that the meat doesn't contain any artificial ingredients like colors, flavors, or preservatives.

11. Season Your Food with Herbs, Spices, and Aromatics

During detoxification, add flavor to your food with cinnamon, ginger, cayenne, garlic, onions, fenugreek, cumin, turmeric, black pepper, parsley, cilantro, vinegar, and citrus zest. These herbs, spices, and aromatics taste good and they're good for you. Several have been shown to reduce fasting blood sugar and insulin levels and improve blood sugar control, including ginger (Rani et al. 2011); cinnamon, cayenne, garlic, onions, and fenugreek (Ballali and Lanciai 2011); turmeric (Madkor, Mansour, and Ramadan 2011); cilantro (Sreelatha and Inbavalli 2012); and parsley (Bolkent et al. 2004). Vinegar consumed with meals (two teaspoons) has been shown to lower blood-sugar levels two hours after eating (Johnston et al. 2010). Vinegar is also a fermented food and supports good digestion. Limonene, a compound found in the essential oils of citrus-fruit peels, can reduce insulin resistance and stimulate detoxification enzymes in the liver (Victor Antony Santiago et al. 2012).

Ginger, cinnamon, and cayenne also promote detoxification by increasing elimination through sweating, and they reduce inflammation in the body (Tilgner 1999). Turmeric also helps detoxify cancer-causing chemicals (Nagabhushan and Bhide 1992), protects against free-radical (oxidative) damage, fights inflammation (Lim et al. 2001), and increases the flow of bile from the liver (Boonjaraspinyo et al. 2011). Turmeric should always be eaten in combination with ground black pepper, as turmeric is poorly absorbed when eaten alone, but black pepper increases its absorption by 2,000 percent (Shoba et al. 1998).

Cumin has been shown to significantly increase levels of anti-oxidants, including glutathione in the liver (Kanter, Coskun, and Gurel 2005). Cilantro also acts as an antioxidant (Sreelatha and Inbavalli 2012), protects the liver against damage from high levels of blood sugar and environmental toxins (Sreelatha, Padma, and Umadevi 2009), and helps remove heavy metals from the body, especially mercury, lead, and aluminum (Omura and Beckman 1995).

If you're not already familiar with these herbs and spices, experiment and learn how to incorporate them into your cooking. An excellent guide is *Healing Spices* by Bharat B. Aggarwal. I like to buy whole spices (like cumin seeds instead of ground cumin) whenever I can and grind them as needed, to keep the medicinal compounds as potent as possible for as long as possible. When it comes to garlic, one of the main medicinal compounds is allicin, and it's formed from an inactive precursor only upon exposure to air. To maximize the benefits of garlic, increase the surface area exposed to air by grating it or by crushing it with a garlic press and then setting it aside for a few minutes to allow the reactions to happen to their fullest extent. Allicin is destroyed by heat, so the less you cook it, the better. Use raw grated garlic whenever you can. On occasions that call for cooking, add garlic to dishes at the end of cooking, and never heat it for more than ten minutes.

Pesticides on Cilantro

Even though cilantro isn't on the Dirty Dozen Plus list, you should avoid it if it isn't organic. The US Department of Agriculture routinely tests produce for pesticides, and their most recent analysis included cilantro (USDA 2011). Researchers tested 184 samples, both domestic (81 percent) and foreign, and they detected pesticides on 94 percent. One pesticide in particular (chlorpyrifros) was found to exceed the limit set by the Environmental Protection Agency by up to 300 percent. Samples also tested positive for thirty-four unapproved pesticides, and washing did not remove them. If you can't find organic cilantro at your farmers' market or in stores, grow your own in your garden or inside a pot on a sunny windowsill.

12. Avoid Food Contact with Plastic or Nonstick Surfaces

Toxic chemicals like BPA, phthalates, and PFCs can migrate from plastic, polystyrene, and nonstick surfaces into foods and beverages and then into our bodies. To avoid these toxins, avoid packaged foods and drinks whenever possible unless they come in glass containers. As an alternative to canned beans, soak dried beans overnight and cook them yourself. You can store cooked beans in glass jars, covered with their cooking liquid, in the fridge or freezer, so you don't have to soak and cook them each time you want to eat them. Buy eggs in cardboard cartons instead of plastic or polystyrene cartons.

Do not drink beverages out of plastic bottles (not even spring water), cups, or travel mugs. Use stainless-steel or glass containers instead. Replace plastic food-storage containers with ceramic or tempered-glass containers and BPA-free lids. Widemouthed canning jars work well for storing dry goods like beans, as well as soups, sauces, and stocks. Replace plastic wrap with unbleached waxed paper, which is nontoxic and biodegradable, or aluminum foil. Eliminate your need for plastic bags by using reusable organic cotton shopping bags. You can learn more about nontoxic food and beverage containers at www.prediabetesdetox.com.

Replace nonstick cookware with cast-iron, stainless-steel, glass, or ceramic cookware. People are often reluctant to give up their nonstick pans because they think that food will stick to cast-iron or stainless steel surfaces. To prevent food from sticking to these types of pans, you don't need large amounts of oil. You just need the correct technique. There are three simple rules: Preheat the pan and the cooking fat until they are hot before you add any food. Only cook foods that are at room temperature, not cold or straight from the fridge. And avoid moving around or flipping the food in the pan prematurely. Allow the food to pull away from the pan on its own, which will happen naturally once it finishes cooking.

When it comes to stainless-steel cookware, look for pots and pans with an aluminum core for even heat distribution and the designation "18/10," which refers to the percentages of chromium and aluminum in the stainless-steel alloy, added for rust resistance and shine.

Oven-safe glass and ceramic baking dishes tend to cook foods faster than metal pans, so compensate by lowering your oven temperature by 25 degrees when baking with glass dishes.

If nonstick pans are your only choice, never preheat them when they are empty, use them only over low heat, never put them in the oven, and discard them as soon as the surface becomes scratched.

You can learn more about nontoxic cookware at www.prediabetes detox.com.

It's also a good idea to limit your use of microwave ovens. They emit radiofrequency radiation that can increase the amount of AGEs in foods (Harvey and French 2000). The damage is dose dependent, so using microwave ovens to warm foods for short periods of time does less damage than using them to cook foods for longer periods of time.

13. Drink Plenty of Filtered Water

Take your weight in pounds and drink half that number in ounces of filtered water every day. For example, a 150-pound person should drink at least seventy-five ounces of water daily. Drinking plenty of water supports the elimination of environmental toxins through the kidneys. Your urine should be a clear light yellow and almost color-less. If it's not, you need to drink more water.

More than fifty million people in the United States drink pol-luted water (EWG 2009a). The same study found that US drinking water contains 315 pollutants and that more than half were not subject to safety guidelines. Forty-nine of the regulated chemicals were found to exceed existing guidelines. You can find out what's in your water with some help from the Environmental Working Group's National Drinking Water Database (find the link at www .prediabetesdetox.com).

To minimize your exposure to toxins in drinking water, use a water filter. Activated carbon filters remove chlorine, lead, mercury, copper, pesticides, solvents, radon, parasites, some volatile organic compounds (VOCs), and bad tastes and odors from tap water. In addition, reverse-osmosis filters remove fluoride, cadmium, asbes-tos, bacteria, arsenic, barium, nitrates, nitrites, and perchlorate. Reverse-osmosis filters use thin membranes and claim to remove 99.97 percent of contaminants 0.3 microns or larger while ultra-HEPA filters reportedly filter out 99.99 percent. Reverse-osmosis filter systems use more water and are more expensive up front, but they are less expensive in the long run. Before you buy any filter, check out the water-filter buying guide from the Environmental

Working Group. (Find a link to the guide at www.prediabetesdetox
.com.) Remember to change the filters regularly.

Filtered water is the best kind of water to drink. If you have a
hard time with this, the next best choice is pure, unflavored sparkling water or sodium-free seltzer water from glass bottles. You can
add your own flavor, if you wish, with fresh sprigs of mint or slices
of citrus fruit or cucumber. Use filtered water for cooking and
making tea.

14. Drink Three or More Cups of Unsweetened Tea Daily

Include three or more cups of hot or cold unsweetened tea in your
daily water intake. All true teas—white, green, oolong, and black—
come from the leaves of the *Camellia sinensis* plant. They contain
powerful antioxidants, including epigallocatechin gallate-3 (or
EGCG), which has been shown to raise levels of glutathione (Na
and Surh 2008), stimulate detoxification pathways in the liver, and
increase elimination of chemicals associated with insulin resistance
and diabetes (Morita, Matsueda, and Iida 1999). EGCG has also
been shown to protect the brain from heavy metals (Mandel et al.
2006).

White tea comes from young leaves that are steamed immediately after harvest and not fermented at all. It contains the highest
concentration of EGCG. Green tea has undergone minimal fermentation and is also high in EGCG, especially Japanese varieties like
matcha, sencha, and gyokuro. Oolong tea is partially fermented, and
black tea is fully fermented. The process of fermentation changes
some of the antioxidants in tea leaves, transforming them into new
compounds (like theaflavins and thearubigins) that also reduce the
risk of diabetes.

To maximize the health benefits of tea, drink it unsweetened
and avoid adding dairy products like cream, as they inactivate the
beneficial compounds. Look for loose tea leaves (or ground tea leaves
in the case of matcha) and use one teaspoon for each cup of water, or
use more if you like a stronger flavor. Sometimes tea (especially

Bottled Water

In the United States, we drink nearly nine billion gallons of bottled water each year, and it costs us almost twelve billion dollars annually, according to the International Bottled Water Association (2008). The Environmental Protection Agency sets standards for tap water from public water systems, but bottled water is not held to these standards. Companies that produce bottled water are not required to disclose information about contaminants or inform customers where the water comes from, whether or not it is purified, or how purification is done.

The Environmental Working Group tested ten popular bottled water brands and found chemical contaminants in every single sample, some exceeding legal limits (EWG 2008). Researchers detected thirty-eight pollutants in total, with an average of eight in each brand, including:

- Bacteria

- Heavy metals like arsenic

- Radioactive elements

- Waste pollutants like caffeine and pharmaceutical drugs

- Fertilizer residues like nitrates and ammonia

- Industrial chemicals like solvents, propellants, and plasticizers

- Chemicals that have been linked to cancer and reproductive problems, like trihalomethanes and bromodichloromethane.

Bottled water costs about nineteen hundred times more than tap water, yet studies show that the two are chemically indistinguishable. And in some cases, bottled water is actually tap water in a bottle. According to the Environmental Working Group, Walmart water was found to be bottled Las Vegas tap water (EWG 2008).

Transporting filtered tap water in reusable stainless-steel or glass containers isn't just better for you; it's also better for the environment. Plastic water bottles are one of the fastest growing sources of garbage, and transporting them across the country and around the world burns massive amounts of fossil fuels, releasing carbon dioxide and other pollution into the environment. "The plastic bottles produced for water require 1.5 million barrels of oil per year, enough to generate electricity for 250,000 homes or fuel 100,000 cars for a year," according to the US Conference of Mayors (2007, 160).

green tea) can cause mild nausea when you drink it on an empty stomach. If this happens to you, add water to dilute the tea, substitute matcha or limit yourself to white tea.

Herbal teas rooibos, dandelion, and ginger aren't made from the *Camellia sinensis* plant, so they aren't true teas, but they also support detoxification and elimination. (Technically, they're infusions, but for the purposes of this book I'll refer to them as teas, for this is how they will be prepared and used.) Rooibos comes from a plant native to South Africa. It's caffeine-free and rich in polyphenols, compounds that act as antioxidants and fight oxidative stress (Scalbert et al. 2005). Studies show that rooibos increases gluthathione levels in the liver (Marnewick et al. 2003), supports phase 2 detoxification, and protects the liver from oxidative damage (Ulicná et al. 2003). Dandelion tea is made from steeping the dried leaves or root of the plant (chapter 4 will go further into its health benefits). As mentioned previously, ginger fights inflammation and increases elimination. Ginger tea can be made from the dried root, but the fresh root, thinly sliced to maximize surface area, makes a more potent and flavorful tea.

Most tea steeping guidelines are designed to optimize flavor, but mine are designed to optimize extraction of beneficial compounds. If a longer infusion makes your tea too bitter for your taste, reduce the steeping time.

Tea	Ideal steeping temperature	Ideal steeping time
Green tea	160°F (when small bubbles start to appear)	five to ten minutes
White tea	175° to 185°F (when strings of bubbles rise to the surface)	four to fifteen minutes
Oolong tea	195°F (almost a full boil)	five to nine minutes
Black tea	203°F (full boil)	three to six minutes
Rooibos	203°F (full boil)	ten-plus minutes
Dandelion	203°F (full boil)	twenty-plus minutes
Ginger	203°F (full boil)	twenty-plus minutes

If coffee doesn't cause you to have anxiety, restlessness, stomach irritation, or problems sleeping, and if you can drink it unsweetened, you can have up to one serving of coffee per day in the morning. Coffee is high in antioxidants and has been shown to protect the liver from toxic chemicals (Ozercan et al. 2006), and some studies have even found it to have blood-sugar and insulin-lowering effects (Psaltopoulou, Ilias, and Alevizaki 2010). If you drink unsweetened coffee, you can have eight ounces of brewed coffee or one shot of espresso each morning, but don't drink it after noon or count it toward your water intake. If you make it yourself, consider adding ground cinnamon to the coffee grounds before brewing. The flavor is lovely, and cinnamon is one of the spices you should be consuming regularly. If you wish, add real cream, preferably organic or from grass-fed cows. If you want a dairy-free alternative, or if you can't find organic cream, you can add fresh homemade nut milk.

Vegetarian Detox Diet

Vegetarians can certainly follow the prediabetes detox diet with some minor modifications. Because plant foods are made mostly of carbohydrates, and animal foods are made mostly of fat and protein, people who only eat plants naturally eat more carbohydrates and less fat and protein. Their challenge during detoxification is to be diligent about getting enough of these nutrients. Good sources of meatless protein include raw nuts, raw nut butters, beans and lentils, tempeh, eggs, and dairy products like cheese, and yogurt.

Vegans, who don't eat any animal products at all, will be missing some amino acids that are essential during detoxification. If you don't eat meat, eggs, or any animal products, you'll want to have at least two servings of protein powder per day to compensate (see chapter 4).

The Soy Debate

It's common for people who don't eat meat to rely on soy as a regular source of protein, but it's not necessarily good for everyone.

Eating Out

The prediabetes detox diet is easiest when you cook your own food. If you have to eat out, plan ahead and follow these guidelines to get the healthiest and most detox-friendly meal possible:

- Pick the restaurant ahead of time and look at the menu online to make sure it will suit your dietary needs.

- Order foods prepared by grilling, steaming, or roasting.

- Skip sauces and dressings unless you know that all of the ingredients are detox friendly.

- Season foods with extra-virgin olive oil and vinegar or freshly squeezed lemon (ask for lemon wedges).

- Follow the same meal formula that you would at home: protein, fat, and fiber with at least 50 percent green vegetables.

- If the only meat available has not been pasture-raised, eat beans, fish, or eggs instead.

- Choose an entrée salad topped with protein if possible.

- Avoid breaded foods, deep-fried dishes, pasta, rice, potatoes, and bread.

- If a bread basket is provided, ask your waitperson to take it away or not to bring it in the first place.

- If your meal comes with starches, ask to substitute them with extra vegetables.

- If you don't see a meal that meets your needs, don't be afraid to ask for what you want, even if it's not on the menu.

- Order plain fresh berries for dessert.

Soy is one of the ten most common food allergens, and reactions may be diverse, but the most common symptoms of soy sensitivity are gas and bloating. If you don't digest soy products well, avoid them. If you're not sure whether you are sensitive to soy, avoid all forms of it during the detox. Then reintroduce it according to the guidelines in chapter 7.

People who do eat soy should follow these five guidelines:

1. Eat organic soy. Always buy soy products that are certified organic to ensure that you aren't ingesting pesticides or genetically modified food.

2. Eat fermented forms. Like other beans, soy contains phytic acid, which can be difficult to digest and may bind to minerals and interfere with their absorption. Fermenting soybeans neutralizes phytic acid and increases their digestibility. It also makes nutrients easier for your body to absorb and utilize and adds live cultures of healthy microorganisms that support good digestion and even help break down pesticides. Fermented forms of soy include tempeh, miso, and tamari.

3. Avoid processed products. Don't eat foods containing soy extracts that may have been removed with toxic chemical solvents. Read labels carefully and stay away from soy protein isolates, soy protein concentrates, textured soy protein, hydrolyzed soy protein, soy flour, soy lecithin, and soybean oil. Avoid soy milk and fake foods like soy meat and soy cheese. Tofu is minimally processed, but it's not fermented, so choose tempeh instead whenever you can. As an alternative to store-bought soy-based veggie burgers, learn to make your own in a food processor using a protein base like tempeh or cooked beans, a binder such as ground nuts or an egg (instead of bread crumbs), and your choice of vegetables, herbs, and spices.

4. Add sea foods. Soy can affect thyroid function in people who are iodine deficient, so supplement soy with iodine-rich foods like sea vegetables (seaweed), fish, and seafood.

5. Use moderation. Soy sensitivity is especially common among people who eat it several times each day. Limit soy consumption to once daily and be sure to incorporate other healthy meatless sources of protein into your diet, like other varieties of beans, lentils, nuts, seeds, eggs, cheese, yogurt, and kefir.

Foods and Beverages to Avoid

These foods should be completely avoided during the prediabetes detox diet:

Fruits

All fruit except for organic whole berries and some citrus fruit (see list of foods to consume).

Jam and jelly

Dried fruit

Fruit juice

Fruit concentrate

Canned fruit

Fruit-based sweeteners

Vegetables

Carrots

Parsnips

Pumpkin

Winter squash

Rutabagas

Sweet potatoes

Potatoes, including potato chips, French fries, and potato starch

Yams

Nonorganic celery

Nonorganic cucumbers

Nonorganic bell peppers

Nonorganic leafy greens

Nonorganic string beans

Nonorganic summer squash

Nonorganic zucchini

Vegetable oil

Nuts, Seeds, Grains, and Legumes

All forms of roasted and toasted nuts, including nut butters, nut oils, and tahini (sesame seed paste)

All whole and processed grains, including white rice, brown rice, basmati rice, jasmine rice, oatmeal, rye, barley, wheat berries, quinoa, spelt, amaranth, millet, kasha, buckwheat, bulgur, kamut, teff, corn, cornstarch, corn syrup, corn chips, durum, farina, semolina, and seitan

Foods made from flour, including bread, pasta, couscous, crackers, bagels, pretzels, bread crumbs, breaded foods, cereals, pastries, cakes, and cookies

Processed soy, including fake meat, fake cheese, soy protein isolates, soy protein concentrates, textured soy protein, and hydrolyzed soy protein

Liquid oils that have not been cold-pressed, including soybean oil, corn oil, canola oil, sunflower oil, safflower oil, cottonseed oil, peanut oil, and vegetable oil

Expeller-Pressed Oils

Expeller-pressed oils are extracted with mechanical force instead of hexane gas, but they're not necessarily cold-pressed. The harder the original substance, the more pressure is required to extract its oil. Higher pressures create more friction between molecules and therefore more heat. Unless the label specifically says that an oil is cold-pressed, assume that it's not. Even organic expeller-pressed oils can contain damaged, inflammatory fatty acids.

Fish and Seafood

Farm-raised species except for rainbow trout, Arctic char, and oysters

Large predatory fish and contaminated seafood, including wild salmon from Washington/Oregon/California, king mackerel, tuna, bluefish, blue crab, Chilean sea bass, flounder, marlin, orange roughy, rockfish, shark, snapper, sturgeon, swordfish, tilefish, walleye, yellow perch, lingcod, and opah

Breaded fish

Processed fish products like fish patties, fish sticks, fish cakes, and fish balls

Meat and Animal Products

Processed meats, including sliced deli meat, hot dogs, pepperoni, salami, bologna, and Spam

Breaded meats

Sausage that isn't homemade

All meat, eggs, and dairy products from animals fed grains or exposed to pesticides, hormones, antibiotics, or other drugs

Charred, smoked, and grilled meats

Egg substitutes

Milk

Ice cream

Processed cheese

Nonorganic, low-fat, and fat-free dairy products

Commercial varieties of kefir, buttermilk, sour cream, cream cheese, and cottage cheese

Flavored or sweetened yogurt

Sweets

All sweetened foods, whether naturally or artificially sweetened

Condiments and Seasonings

Sweetened condiments, including ketchup, relish, barbeque sauce, hoisin sauce, chutney, and store-bought salad dressing (make your own instead)

Margarine, vegetable-oil spreads, and other butter alternatives

Beverages

All naturally or artificially sweetened beverages, including soft drinks, soda, diet soda, energy drinks, sports drinks, and flavored water

Juice

Cow's milk and store-bought milk alternatives, including rice milk, soy milk, almond milk, and coconut milk packaged as a beverage

Nondairy creamers

Alcohol

Other

Processed and manufactured foods

Deep-fried foods

Any foods that you are or may be allergic or sensitive to, including dairy products

Foods and Beverages to Consume

During the prediabetes detox diet, the following foods may be consumed in unlimited but reasonable quantities unless otherwise noted:

Vegetables

Artichokes

Asparagus

Avocados

Beets (limited to a half-cup serving up to two times per day)

Beet greens

Organic bell peppers

Broccoli

Brussels sprouts

Organic celery

Cabbage

Cauliflower

Organic chard

Organic collard greens

Organic cucumber

Eggplant

Endive

Organic kale

Leeks

Mushrooms

Organic mustard greens

Okra

Onions

Olives

Peppers

Pickles

Radishes

Organic salad greens

Sauerkraut

Sea vegetables (including hijiki, kombu, nori, wakame)

Organic spinach

Organic string beans

Organic summer squash

Organic zucchini

Fruit

Organic whole berries only, fresh or frozen and unsweetened, without sauce or syrup (limited to a half-cup serving once per day)

Whole citrus fruit, excluding grapefruit (limited to one piece or a half-cup serving once per day)

Organic citrus zest (unlimited)

Lemon juice and lime juice (unlimited)

Fermented Foods

Vinegar

Yogurt with live cultures

Aged and ripened cheeses (avoid processed cheeses)

Cultured butter

Sauerkraut

Kimchi

Umeboshi

Lacto-fermented pickles, capers, and olives

Tempeh, miso, and tamari

Fish sauce

Cacao nibs

Nuts, Seeds, and Beans

Raw nuts (limited to a half cup at a time, up to two times per day), especially raw walnuts, macadamia nuts, and almonds

Raw nut butters like almond butter (limited to two table-spoons at a time, up to two times per day)

Homemade nut milks (made with raw soaked nuts and filtered water)

Raw seeds, especially ground flaxseeds and chia seeds

Unsweetened coconut (fresh or dried), pure coconut milk, coconut water

Organic fermented soy products, including tempeh, miso, and tamari

Whole beans, presoaked or sprouted and slow cooked (limited to a half-cup serving up to two times a day), including lentils, black beans, butter beans, kidney beans, navy beans, pinto beans, white beans, black-eyed peas, chickpeas (garbanzo beans), and fava beans

Fish and Seafood

Wild salmon from Alaska

Sablefish from the United States or Canada

Herring

Atlantic mackerel from Canada (avoid Spanish and King mackerel)

Pacific sardines from the United States

Pacific halibut from Alaska or Canada

Anchovies

Rainbow trout

Arctic char

Oysters

Clams

Scallops

Dungeness crab (avoid blue crab)

Wild-caught spiny lobster

Squid (calamari)

Haddock

Atlantic pollock

Wild-caught pink shrimp

Wild-caught spot prawns

Meat and Animal Products

Eat only products from pasture-raised and grass-fed animals and wild game:

Whole eggs

Whole-milk organic dairy products, including yogurt, heavy cream, butter, and aged and ripened cheeses from cows, sheep, and goats (optional)

Lamb

Duck

Chicken

Turkey

Pheasant

Game Birds

Ostrich

Buffalo

Venison

Elk

Beef

Boar

Pork

Rabbit

Organ meats like liver, sweetbreads, gizzards, heart, kidneys, tongue, and tripe

Bone marrow

Bone broth

Sweets

Organic whole berries

Whole citrus fruit, except grapefruit

85 percent dark chocolate (limited to one ounce per day)

Stevia (limited to one gram per day)

Condiments and Seasonings

Cold-pressed oils: extra-virgin olive, coconut, walnut, flax-seed (store them in the refrigerator)

Unsweetened vinegars

Sea salt

Peppercorns (ground pepper)

Ginger

Garlic

Shallots

Herbs

Spices

Kimchee

Umeboshi paste

Salsa

Hot sauce (if it's just chili peppers, vinegar, and salt)

Pesto

Tapenade

Real mayonnaise

Homemade Dijon-style mustard

Remember to check food labels on purchased products for any unwanted ingredients.

Beverages

Filtered water

Hot or cold unsweetened tea: white, green, oolong, rooibos, dandelion, and ginger

One cup of unsweetened coffee per day (optional), either eight ounces of brewed coffee or one shot of espresso, regular or decaffeinated by the Swiss-water method (chemical-free)

chapter 4
Prediabetes Detox Supplements

Supplementation is an important part of the prediabetes detox program, for it ensures that your body will be getting adequate support for the mobilization, detoxification, and elimination of environmental chemicals. Everything that happens in the body comes down to chemistry, and when the nutrients that drive certain reactions are missing, those reactions just don't happen. During detox, if you don't get the necessary vitamins, minerals, antioxidants, and amino acids, toxins that have been mobilized can be put back into storage, retoxifying your body instead of detoxifying it.

In an ideal world, the vitamins, minerals, and antioxidants we need would come from food. But in the real world, it's almost impossible to get all of the nutrients our bodies need from our diets alone. Modern-day lifestyles, prescription medications, and chronic illnesses increase our needs for nutrients, but foods today are significantly less nutritious than the wild ones that were available to our ancestors. Industrial-farming methods like growing monocultures and using chemical fertilizers have depleted the nutrients in soil, and if these nutrients aren't available, plants can't absorb them. We've selected and engineered plant species for their appearance and shelf life, not for their nutritional content. We pick fruits and vegetables before they're ripe (unripe produce has significantly less nutrients than mature produce) and ship them long distances, which depletes nutrient stores even further. Air pollution and rising levels of carbon dioxide in the atmosphere also reduce the nutritional content of the plants we eat (Chai et al. 2011). Food-manufacturing methods destroy vitamins, and a large part of the foods we eat have been processed. And no longer do most people in the United States consume nutrient-rich organ meats on a regular basis.

Supplements can compensate for what's missing, so think of them as health insurance. These supplements are recommended for everyone as part of the prediabetes detox program:

- A multivitamin/mineral formula

- Extra vitamin C: 2,000 milligrams two to three times per day

- Extra magnesium: 400 milligrams two times per day

- Vitamin D: 1,000 to 2,000 international units (IU) per day

- Alpha lipoic acid: 600 milligrams two times per day

- Omega-3 fats: 2,000 milligrams of DHA and EPA (combined total) of fish or algae oil

- Liver-supportive herbs like milk thistle, dandelion, and burdock

- Probiotics: 10 billion microorganisms per day

Additionally, I recommend taking green-tea capsules if you're not drinking enough tea, and I recommend using a protein powder if you're following a vegan diet.

It's a good idea to take these supplements at the very beginning of meals, just before your first bite.

Combining them with food will ensure that the fat-soluble supplements will be properly absorbed (because each of your meals will contain healthy fat). Sometimes minerals or plant extracts can cause nausea or upset when taken on an empty stomach, so taking them with food also prevents this problem. If you have difficulty swallowing capsules, open them up and stir the contents into water or a small amount of plain yogurt.

This chapter will discuss each of these supplements in detail and give you guidelines for selecting supplements. If you want information on the specific products that I recommend for my patients and take myself, visit www.prediabetesdetox.com.

Multivitamin/Mineral Supplements

Look for multivitamin/mineral formulas that contain vitamins A, C, D, E, and K; B vitamins including thiamine (B1), riboflavin (B2), niacin (B3), pantothenic acid (B5), pyridoxine (B6), biotin, folic acid, and cobalamin (B12); minerals including calcium, magnesium, potassium, zinc, and iron (if you need it); and trace minerals including chromium, selenium, manganese, copper, molybdenum, boron, and vanadium. Some of these nutrients also act as antioxidants, including vitamin C, vitamin E, vitamin A, selenium, and zinc.

To separate the good products from the bad and find one that best meets your individual needs, you will want to consider several factors.

Mineral Chelates

MVM supplements contain minerals in *chelated* form. This means that they are bound to an amino acid that allows them to be absorbed by the body. Some mineral chelates are more *bioavailable* than others, which means that they are more easily digested and absorbed. For example, calcium citrate, calcium malate, and calcium aspartate are more bioavailable and better tolerated than calcium carbonate, a cheaper form of calcium that can be difficult to digest. Calcium carbonate can also be constipating, and higher doses are required for enough of the mineral to be absorbed. Citrate, malate, and aspartate forms take up more space inside capsules, and they are more costly to produce, so the MVM formulas that use them are often more expensive and require more capsules per serving to get a full daily dose of nutrients (often six per day), but it's worth the extra expense.

Chromium

When it comes to chromium, look for a MVM formula that contains this mineral in picolinate or polynicotinate form. These are the only forms of chromium that effectively lower fasting glucose levels, decrease hemoglobin A1C, increase insulin sensitivity, reduce free-radical production, and protect the liver and kidneys from damage (Preuss et al. 2008). Make sure you're getting at least two hundred micrograms of chromium picolinate or chromium polynicotinate per day.

Iron

Certain people need to supplement iron, including pregnant women, growing children, women who menstruate, and people who have confirmed low levels, which isn't uncommon in individuals following vegetarian and vegan diets. If you're unsure, your doctor can order a simple blood test that will determine if your levels are low. Don't take it if you don't need it, because too much iron can increase insulin resistance and the risk for cardiovascular disease. If you do need it, choose a MVM formula with iron citrate, iron aspartate, iron succinate, or iron fumarate, for these forms are the most bioavailable and least constipating. Adult men and postmenopausal women who eat meat usually don't need extra iron.

Beta Carotene

Anyone who has a history of smoking should avoid MVMs with vitamin A in the form of beta carotene. In this population, beta carotene has been correlated with an increased risk of lung cancer and prostate cancer.

E Vitamins

Vitamin E naturally exists in eight related compounds: four tocotrienols and four tocopherols, each designated alpha, beta, gamma, and delta. Men should avoid MVMs with D-alpha-tocopherol as the only form of vitamin E, for it has been associated with an increased risk of prostate cancer.

Activated Vitamins

For some people, taking the most active forms of certain vitamins is most effective, including the D3 form of vitamin D, the pyridoxyl-5-phosphate form of B6, the methylcobalamin form of B12, and the methylfolate form of folic acid.

Copper

Long-term supplementation of zinc can lead to copper deficiency if you don't take both copper and zinc, so most people should have both in their MVM. Avoid copper in the form of cupric oxide, as it's very poorly absorbed. People who have cancer should avoid copper completely.

Digestive Enzymes

Digestive enzymes like amylase (to digest carbohydrates), lipase (to digest fats), and protease (to digest proteins) are added to some MVM formulas to help you break down your food better. They can be helpful for certain people and for short periods of time, but digestive enzymes aren't a good idea for everyone, and they don't belong in MVM formulas. Taken regularly, they can cause your pancreas to become less efficient at producing your body's own enzymes. If you're having problems with digestion, talk to your naturopathic doctor about possible underlying causes before you supplement digestive enzymes.

Extras

Coenzyme Q10 is a powerful antioxidant and a critical part of producing energy inside every single cell. It's not included in all

MVM formulas, but it's a good idea if you are on a blood sugar–lowering, blood pressure–lowering, cholesterol-lowering, or antidepressant medication, if you are low on energy, if you have heart disease or are at a high risk of developing heart disease, if you are vegetarian or vegan, or if you are over the age of fifty (because our bodies naturally produce less CoQ10 as we age). Other extras I like to see are alpha-lipoic acid, green tea, and turmeric.

Additives

Avoid supplements with artificial colors or flavors, which are common in chewable, powdered, and liquid supplements. Also avoid formulas with fillers, binders, flowing agents, coatings, preservatives, food dyes, and pro-inflammatory oils. Specific ingredients to avoid include soybean oil, magnesium stearate, stearic acid, silicon dioxide, and titanium dioxide.

Manufacturer

Some supplements have been found to be contaminated with harmful substances like lead, mercury, cadmium, and arsenic and pesticide residues. Only buy products from companies that your naturopathic doctor has recommended or that meet the criteria I explain at the end of this chapter.

Always take MVM supplements with food, for they contain fat-soluble vitamins that you otherwise won't absorb. Split up the total daily dose into two or three servings and spread them throughout the day. For example, if a full dose is six capsules, take two capsules three times per day (with breakfast, lunch, and dinner) or three capsules two times per day (with breakfast and dinner).

Remember that MVM supplements aren't a substitute for a healthy diet. Lots of nutrients exist in nature not as single molecules but as families of related molecules that work synergistically together but aren't found in supplements. MVMs are good insurance that you're getting the basics, but also take advantage of nutrients in whole foods to get the extras.

Protein Powder

Protein powders are optional during detoxification unless you follow a vegan diet. If this is the case, you'll need at least two servings of protein powder per day to meet your amino acid requirement. Some protein powders do double duty as MVM supplements. If you use a protein powder to make a smoothie every day and it has a full range of vitamins and minerals, you don't need a separate MVM supplement. Avoid protein powders made from soy, and look for products free of added sugar, artificial sweeteners, and artificial flavors.

The protein powder I recommend most often to my patients is made from a combination of hemp seeds, peas, and rice. Hemp seeds add omega-3 fats, and peas are especially high in protein compared to other plant foods. It's hypoallergenic and free of wheat, gluten, dairy, egg, soy, corn, yeast, nuts, sugar, artificial sweeteners, colors, and preservatives. It also contains the full spectrum of nutrient cofactors needed for detoxification and some extras like green tea and milk thistle (which you'll read more about later in this chapter). Visit www.prediabetesdetox.com for more information on protein powders like this one.

Whey protein powder is another good option for detox, for it boosts levels of glutathione in the liver and decreases cortisol, a hormone that increases blood sugar and insulin levels (Markus et al. 2000). Whey is a protein found in milk and in the liquid that separates from yogurt (so always stir it back in instead of pouring it off). It provides a good amount of amino acids and about twenty-three grams of protein per serving, but whey doesn't contain any fiber. It's also missing the vitamins and minerals found in other protein powders, so whey protein needs to be taken with a separate MVM supplement.

Whey is removed when milk is made into cheese, so if you have an adverse reaction to milk but not to cheese, then you are not allergic or sensitive to whey. If you react to both milk and cheese, you may be allergic or sensitive to whey and should avoid this protein powder. If you experience gas or bloating, discontinue using it and switch to a dairy-free protein powder.

Because whey protein is an animal product, quality is very important. Look for a whey protein that comes from grass-fed or pasture-raised cows, is processed without high temperatures that can change the nature of its amino acids, and is free of lactose, added sugar, artificial sweeteners, and artificial flavors.

Extra Vitamin C

I recommend taking extra vitamin C, for it helps the liver process toxins and excrete them from the body. Along with vitamin E, vitamin C has also been shown to protect against damage induced by air pollution (Gomes et al. 2011).

During detoxification, I recommend taking at least two thousand milligrams of vitamin C two times per day with meals. Because high doses of vitamin C can cause loose stools, you should start with a lower dose of five hundred milligrams twice per day and gradually increase in five hundred milligram increments to bowel tolerance. If you smoke or live in an urban area, take at least two thousand milligrams three times per day if you tolerate it (and stop smoking immediately). If your stools become too loose, decrease your dosage until they normalize.

The body uses vitamin C best when taken in its natural form, so look for a product that contains bioflavonoids. If you have a sensitive stomach, you should take a buffered form of vitamin C. Otherwise, vitamin C is safe and usually well tolerated.

More Magnesium

Magnesium is the fourth most abundant mineral in the body, and most people in the United States don't get enough. According to the National Health and Nutrition Examination Survey, 68 percent of US adults consume less than the recommended daily allowance (King et al. 2005). You need even more magnesium during detoxification, during periods of stress, and if you have a chronic illness like prediabetes. Magnesium helps transport glucose across cell membranes, activates vitamin D, and plays a part in more than three hundred enzyme systems throughout the body, including the ones in the liver used for detoxification and those attached to adipose cells that release fatty acids and stored toxins. Chronic magnesium deficiency has been associated with insulin resistance and diabetes (Chaudhary, Sharma, and Bansal 2010) while a high intake of magnesium is associated with protection against diabetes (Villegas et al. 2009).

Most MVM formulas contain some magnesium, usually one hundred milligrams, which is a good start, but it's not enough. I recommend taking an additional four hundred milligrams of magnesium two times per day with meals. If you have normal or loose stools, take magnesium glycinate. If you tend toward constipation, take magnesium citrate. Avoid magnesium gluconate, magnesium carbonate, magnesium oxide, and magnesium sulfate.

Like vitamin C, high doses of magnesium can cause loose stools, so it's best to start with a lower dose and increase it gradually. Begin by taking two hundred milligrams twice per day or four hundred milligrams once per day for two to three days, and then increase to 400 milligrams twice per day. If you experience stools that are too loose, decrease your dose to bowel tolerance. Gas and bloating may occur initially, but these symptoms should be temporary, and within a few days your stools should be more moist and easier to pass. Otherwise, magnesium supplements are generally safe and well tolerated.

Vitamin D

If tests show that your vitamin D level is at least thirty-five nanograms per milliliter, I recommend taking 1,000 IU of vitamin D3 (the active form) each day. If your level is below 35 nanograms per milliliter, I recommend taking 2,000 IU of vitamin D3 each day. (If your vitamin D level exceeds normal values, don't take any at all.) In people with high blood sugar and low vitamin D, taking 2,000 IU per day has been shown to improve the function of insulin-producing cells in the pancreas and to slow the rise of hemoglobin A1C (Mitri et al. 2011).

Because vitamin D is a fat-soluble vitamin, it must be taken with some form of fat to be properly absorbed, so take it with meals. It's important not to take too much, because fat-soluble vitamins can accumulate in the body, unlike water-soluble vitamins such as vitamin C, which are easily eliminated by the kidneys. Vitamin D is well tolerated in doses below 10,000 IU per day, but taking too much can damage your bones and organs over time, notably the kidneys. Symptoms of excess vitamin D include constipation, fatigue, lack of appetite, irritability, muscle weakness, vomiting, and dehydration. Vitamin D increases the amount of calcium in the blood (because it plays an important role in bone metabolism), and high levels can prompt the formation of kidney stones. So far, studies using higher amounts of vitamin D haven't shown bigger benefits, so don't take more than 2,000 IU of vitamin D per day unless directed by your doctor.

Besides taking vitamin D as a supplement, it's important to get a daily dose of sunshine, which stimulates the body's own production of vitamin D in the skin. Exactly how much vitamin D your skin makes depends on several different factors: how far you live from the equator, the season of year, the color of your skin (darker skin tones contain more melanin, which blocks radiation from the sun), your age (the older you get, the less vitamin D you make), and how much time you spend in the sun.

Given all of these factors, it's hard to make one recommendation that fits all people, but in general I recommend exposing your skin to sunlight for at least ten to twenty minutes each day. The best time is early morning, when the sun's rays are least intense and least likely to increase your risk for skin cancer. The benefits of sunlight extend beyond vitamin D to normalizing hormones and neurotransmitters that help regulate appetite, blood sugar, and fat storage. Avoid prolonged sun exposure, and if you're outside during the middle of the day, wear a good-quality sunscreen, or better yet, stay in the shade. (See www.prediabetesdetox.com for sunscreen recommendations.)

Alpha-Lipoic Acid

Alpha lipoic acid (or ALA), sometimes called *lipoic acid*, is an antioxidant naturally produced by the body. It's inside every cell, although the highest concentrations are found inside liver cells. ALA is important for detoxification and for reversing prediabetes. Studies show that it neutralizes free radicals, activates phase 2 detoxification, and improves blood sugar balance (Shay et al. 2009); increases levels of glutathione and vitamin C, helps excrete heavy metals, and makes cells more sensitive to insulin (Singh and Jialal 2008); and reduces inflammation (Poh and Goh 2009).

Our natural production of ALA declines as we age and whenever we're sick, so I recommend taking it as a supplement during detoxification and until blood sugar levels normalize. Alpha lipoic acid in supplement form is safe and well tolerated.

Omega-3 Fats

Omega-3 fatty acids are essential for detoxification and for reversing prediabetes. They reduce inflammation in the body, and studies show that DHA and EPA improve blood sugar control (Sartorelli et al. 2010) and insulin sensitivity (Flachs et al. 2009). It's a good idea to get them through your diet by eating nontoxic species of fish and seafood, but during detox you'll need a supplement too. Because so many species of fish and marine animals are now contaminated with toxic environmental chemicals, the quality of fish oil is extremely important. While there are no standards for fish oil quality in the United States, international standards do exist. The Norwegian Medicinal Standard (NMS) and the European Pharmacopoeia Standard (EPS) both set maximum allowances for heavy metals, dioxins, PCBs, and peroxides.

When you're shopping for fish oil, look for products that meet these criteria:

- The manufacturer meets NMS and EPS standards.

- The fish oil is processed without chemicals or excess heat (to maintain the integrity of the fatty acids).

- The fatty acids exist in the natural triglyceride form.

- The manufacturer controls fish oil for freshness (measured by markers called *peroxide* and *anisidine*).

- The manufacturer uses only sustainably harvested fish to make its products.

Fish oil can be found in liquid or capsule form. Liquid forms are usually less expensive than capsules, and they can also be easier to digest. Capsules are easier to transport if you take your fish oil away from home, but some products require taking up to eight capsules per day to get a therapeutic dose. Whether you choose liquid or capsules, always store fish oil in the fridge. (Remember that those fragile unsaturated fatty acids easily oxidize in the presence of heat and light.) Capsules can even be kept in the freezer and swallowed frozen. And if you take your capsules away from home, take only as much as you need out of the fridge or freezer.

Take a combined total of at least two thousand milligrams of DHA and EPA each day during detoxification. Read the label and do the math to determine how many capsules or teaspoons you'll need.

Aside from sensitivity and allergic reactions to fish, these oils are well tolerated. Some of my patients report a fishy aftertaste, but this problem is easily solved by taking frozen fish oil capsules at the very beginning of meals or just before bed (it's okay to take fish oil without food). Other negative side effects are uncommon, but when they do occur, they're usually gastrointestinal in nature, like nausea and diarrhea. Taking fish oil long-term can deplete vitamin E, so small amounts of vitamin E are often added to fish oils.

Fish oil helps prevent blood from getting too sticky and forming clots (coagulating), but it doesn't cause excessive bleeding, and placebo-controlled, randomized, double-blind studies show that it doesn't interfere with anticoagulant medications (Bender et al. 1998).

If you can't take fish oil—either because you don't consume animal products or because you're allergic or sensitive to fish—the next best thing is getting EPA and DHA from algae. It's not as concentrated, so you'll likely have to take more of it to get two thousand milligrams of EPA and DHA daily.

Liver-Supportive Herbs

Plants were the first medicines, and their use dates back to the Neanderthals (who disappeared between twenty-four and thirty thousand years ago). As modern medicine evolved, scientists used plants to make pharmaceutical drugs by isolating specific constituents and manufacturing synthetic versions. Unlike pharmaceutical medications, botanical or herbal medicines are made from whole plants, so they can contain hundreds of different compounds and exert many different effects in the body. Because these compounds complement each other, side effects are less common. Botanical medicines can be grouped into categories based on the actions they have in our bodies, and several categories are useful during detoxification:

- *Antioxidants* that support detoxification pathways in the liver

- *Choleretics* that stimulate production of bile (remember that bile transports toxins from the liver to the intestines, where they can be eliminated with the stool)

- *Cholagogues* that stimulate the release of bile

- *Hepatoprotectives* that protect liver cells from toxin-induced damage

- *Hypoglycemics* and *antihyperglycemics* that support detoxification by lowering blood sugar levels and helping the body to burn fat and release stored toxins

- *Diuretics* that promote elimination by increasing urine output

- *Laxatives* that promote elimination through evacuation of the bowels

Botanical medicines can interact with pharmaceutical medications, so if you're taking a prescription drug, you should talk to your doctor before taking herbal supplements. If your doctor is not trained in the use of botanical medicines, find a naturopathic doctor.

In the same way that people can have allergies or sensitivities to certain foods or prescription medications, people may have allergies or sensitivities to certain herbs. It's not common, but it's possible, and symptoms usually include gastrointestinal upset and skin irritation. It's also possible to have reactions to fillers, binders, preservatives, or other additives in supplements, so make sure that you are using botanical medicines from reputable manufacturers. You'll find criteria at the end of this chapter. If you experience adverse effects while using botanical medicines, discontinue using them.

There are lots of herbs that can support detoxification, but the three most beneficial for people with prediabetes are milk thistle, dandelion, and burdock.

Milk Thistle

Milk thistle (*Silybum marianum*) is an herb with antioxidant, hepatoprotective, and mild laxative properties. It can boost glutathione, prevent free-radical damage, protect cells against toxin-induced damage, and improve liver function (Wellington and Jarvis 2001). It's particularly useful for people with prediabetes, as it also has hypoglycemic properties. Milk thistle has been shown to lower fasting glucose levels and improve insulin resistance in people with high blood sugar (Velussi et al. 1997). Milk thistle is generally safe and well tolerated. Look for a product that is standardized to contain 70 to 80 percent silymarin, and take two hundred to four hundred milligrams per day.

Dandelion

Dandelion (*Taraxacum officinalis*) has antioxidant, anti-inflammatory, hepatoprotective, and antiglycemic activity in the body. It also acts as a choleretic, cholagogue, diuretic, and mild laxative. Dandelion is generally safe and well tolerated in doses up to eight thousand milligrams per day, but you won't need to take that much. During detoxification, you should take five hundred to one thousand milligrams per day. Because dandelion can prevent blood from clotting, it should only be combined with blood-thinning medications under the supervision of a doctor.

Burdock

Burdock (*Arctium lappa*) is an antioxidant and anti-inflammatory agent. It has cholagogue, choleretic, hepatoprotective, diuretic, and mild laxative properties. Some studies also suggest that burdock has hypoglycemic activity (Chan et al. 2011). In Asia, burdock root is added to soups, and the young leaves are often eaten cooked. As a supplement, burdock is generally safe and well tolerated in doses up to eighteen thousand milligrams per day, aside from minor stomach upset associated with high doses. For detoxification, you should take five hundred to one thousand milligrams per day.

Herbs in Combination

These single herbs can be used for detoxification, but they are best used in combination. The formula I use most often in my practice combines milk thistle (50 milligrams per capsule), dandelion (150 milligrams per capsule), and burdock (150 milligrams per capsule), and I recommend that my patients take two capsules twice a day. Visit www.prediabetesdetox.com for more information.

Green Tea

For people who have a hard time drinking enough tea every day, it's a good idea to have green tea capsules on hand. Look for a decaffeinated supplement with a high concentration of EGCG (70 percent) and take five hundred milligrams per day with meals. Taken on an empty stomach, green tea can cause mild nausea.

Probiotics

Beneficial bacteria are essential for good health and especially important for people with prediabetes and those undergoing detoxification. Almost everyone can benefit from probiotic supplementation. Recurrent use of increasingly harsh antibiotics to treat increasingly resistant bacteria, misuse of antibiotics to treat viral infections, consumption of animals treated with antibiotics, contamination of drinking water with antibiotics, and excessive use of antimicrobial chemicals in processed food, hand sanitizers, and household cleaners—all of these factors have altered the ecology of the digestive tract, impairing our abilities to digest and absorb nutrients.

Take about ten billion organisms, or colony-forming units (CFU), per day. If you've taken antibiotics recently, you should take one hundred billion per day for at least two months. Look for a product with several different species of *Lactobacillus* and *Bifidobacterium*, notable *Bifidobacterium Lactis*, shown to improve insulin sensitivity (Vrieze et al. 2012). Some probiotics also contain *prebiotics*, which are complex sugars like inulin, lactulose or fructo-oligosaccharides (FOS) that stimulate the growth of beneficial bacteria. If your supplement does not contain prebiotics, take it with prebiotic-rich foods like ground flaxseeds, artichokes, asparagus, onions, garlic, and/or beans.

Probiotics are generally safe and well tolerated. Side effects are rare and usually limited to mild digestive disturbances such as gas and bloating, which are usually side effects of added prebiotics. If this happens to you, switch to prebiotic-free probiotics.

Probiotics need to be refrigerated to maintain viable and stable live cultures. (Even if the label says that a product need not be refrigerated, keep it in the fridge anyway whenever possible.) If you can, buy products that have been kept cool, either refrigerated in stores or shipped with a cold pack.

Supplement Schedule

As long as you are getting the full doses of the recommended supplements, you can incorporate them into your day however you wish. This is one example of how your daily supplement regimen could look:

With Breakfast

- Multivitamin: 2 capsules

- Extra vitamin C: 2,000 milligrams

- Extra magnesium: 400 milligrams

- Alpha lipoic acid: 600 milligrams

- Herbal formula: 2 capsules

With Lunch

- Multivitamin: 2 capsules

- Extra vitamin C: 2,000 milligrams

- Vitamin D: 1,000–2,000 international units

- Omega-3 fats: 2,000 milligrams of EPA + DHA

- Probiotics: ten billion microorganisms

With Dinner

- Multivitamin: 2 capsules

- Extra vitamin C: 2,000 milligrams

- Extra magnesium: 400 milligrams

- Alpha lipoic acid: 600 milligrams

- Herbal formula: 2 capsules

Heavy Metal Detox

Supplements for heavy metal detoxification deserve special mention. Unlike other environmental toxins, heavy metals like mercury and cadmium can be stored inside connective tissues like bones and inside organs like the brain. Special agents called *chelators* are required to remove them. Chelating agents have the ability to bind to heavy metals, release them from their storage sites, and escort them out of the body. These include DMSA (dimercaptosuccinic acid), DMPS (2,3-dimercapto-1-propanesulfonic acid), and EDTA (ethylenediaminetetraacetic acid). One natural substance, an amino acid called N-acetyle-L-cysteine (or NAC), can increase the excretion of methyl mercury (the form found in fish and seafood), but it's most effective when used in combination with DMSA (Flora and Pachauri 2010). These medicines should only be taken under the care of an experienced physician, who can test you for heavy-metal toxicity and monitor your liver and kidney function before and during treatment.

Treating Constipation

If you're not having daily bowel movements, this must be corrected before you start detoxification. Constipation can be caused by a diet low in fiber, mineral imbalances, dehydration, stress, or lack of exercise. Less common causes of constipation include the use of certain medications and illnesses affecting the digestive tract or the nerves that regulate it.

Because humans cannot digest fiber, it adds bulk to the stool and passes through the body without being absorbed. A bulky stool is important in that it puts pressure on the walls of the intestines, which stimulates peristalsis, the contractions of the smooth muscles that push food through the digestive tract. If you're not eating enough fiber, your stools will be small and may pass through more slowly. If you don't drink enough water, your stools will be dry and difficult to pass, even if you are eating enough fiber.

Stools can also become dry and difficult to pass if you're not getting enough magnesium or if you're getting too much calcium. Calcium is needed for the muscles in your digestive tract to contract, and magnesium is necessary for them to relax. Too much calcium and not enough magnesium cause food to pass more slowly through the gut, allowing too much water to be absorbed, which makes stools dry. (Too much magnesium causes the opposite problem: food passes too quickly through the digestive tract and not enough water is absorbed, which makes stools loose and watery.) An imbalance of calcium and magnesium is common when people take calcium supplements without an equal amount of magnesium.

Stress and a sedentary lifestyle can also contribute to constipation. Stress increases the body's need for magnesium, making a deficiency more likely. Exercise can help manage stress, but it's also important for bowel health. People who exercise are much less likely to be constipated than those who don't exercise, and increasing physical activity can reverse constipation.

It's no coincidence that the prediabetes detox calls for eating a diet high in fluids and fiber, supplementing magnesium, getting plenty of exercise, and managing stress. These activities are as important for detoxification as they are for maintaining regular bowel movements.

If you're not having at least one bowel movement every day, follow these steps before you start the detox program:

1. If you have a gastrointestinal disorder or nerve problem, or if you're taking a medication that is causing constipation, address these issues with your doctor.

2. Drink plenty of filtered water every day unless your doctor has told you otherwise. Take your weight in pounds and drink half that number in ounces every day.

3. Make fibrous green vegetables at least half of every meal. Fibrous vegetables include leafy greens, the cruciferous vegetables described in chapter 3, and other nonstarchy vegetables like artichokes, asparagus, bell peppers, celery, cucumbers, eggplant, green beans, green peas, okra, sauerkraut, tomatoes, yellow summer squash, and zucchini.

4. Consume two tablespoons of ground flaxseeds every day.

5. Exercise for at least one hour five times a week. (See chapter 5 for exercise guidelines.) If you are not already exercising, get permission from your doctor first.

6. Manage stress effectively. (See chapter 5 for recommendations.)

Following these steps is often enough to resolve constipation, but if it's not enough for you, consider adding aloe vera juice. When the juice is made from the inner fillet, aloe vera is a mild laxative.

Aloe vera made from the whole leaf is a stronger laxative because it contains natural compounds called *anthraquinones*. Aloe vera has also been shown to lower fasting blood sugar in people with high blood sugar (Ghannam et al. 1986).

Food-grade aloe vera juice is available at most health food stores. Take one-quarter cup (two ounces) of aloe vera juice before meals or added to smoothies one to three times per day as needed. Both forms of aloe vera (whole leaf and inner fillet) are generally safe and well tolerated for short-term use. If you experience abdominal cramping or diarrhea while taking it, decrease your dose to bowel tolerance.

If you are using whole-leaf aloe vera, limit your use to eight ounces per day for ten consecutive days. When used over the long term, it can deplete potassium, which can lead to muscle weakness and make constipation worse. An overdose can lead to gastrointestinal distress and kidney inflammation. Natural anthraquinones can interact with certain medications. If you're taking a medicine for your heart, talk to your doctor before using whole leaf aloe vera and get your doctor's permission before undertaking a detox program.

If you suffer from chronic constipation, you may want to consider colon hydrotherapy, or *colonics*. It's just what it sounds like, a water treatment for your colon. Performed by a trained professional, colonics cleanse the colon by flushing it with water. This stimulates bile ducts to dilate, increasing the elimination of toxin-laden bile from the liver. Start with two treatments per week for two weeks, then one or two treatments per week as needed.

Colonics can be continued during detoxification, and they have been shown to increase the elimination of toxins (Crinnion 2010). Consider taking a sauna before colon hydrotherapy to increase toxin elimination during the treatment. After the treatment, consume plenty of foods rich in electrolytes and take a probiotic supplement for at least ten days. If you have gastrointestinal health concerns, talk to your doctor before using colon hydrotherapy. Do not use colon hydrotherapy if you have abdominal pain, high blood pressure, or congestive heart failure, or if you've ever had colon surgery.

Once you're having at least one bowel movement per day, you can start the detox program. If you've followed all of these recommendations for treating constipation, and you still aren't having at least one bowel movement per day, you should consult with a naturopathic physician, for there may be other underlying problems that need to be addressed.

Selecting Supplements

Supplements are big business, and some manufacturers cut corners to increase profits. But quality always suffers. If you don't have a naturopathic physician to make recommendations, opt for capsules over tablets, which can contain binders that prevent important ingredients from being fully digested and absorbed. Also avoid liquids, powders, and chewable forms that contain added sweetners, flavors, colors, and preservatives. Look for products that list the following information on the label:

- The name and address of the manufacturer

- A lot number or batch number

- An expiration date

- The scientific name, quantity, and part of any plant ingredient

To ensure that an independent lab has tested products, look for seals from the United States Pharmacopeia, the National Nutritional Foods Association, Consumer Lab, or National Sanitation Foundation International. Such certification guarantees that supplements contain what they are labeled to contain. Be aware, however, that it doesn't ensure that manufacturers started with the highest quality raw ingredients or tested them in clinical trials.

Just One Piece

During detoxification, supplements provide your body with the tools it needs to mobilize and eliminate toxins from the body and effectively regulate blood sugar and insulin. Like diet, supplements are just one piece of the detox puzzle. Another important component is lifestyle, which is the focus of the next chapter.

chapter 5

Prediabetes Detox Lifestyle

A healthy lifestyle is just as important as a healthy diet when it comes to detoxification, reversing prediabetes, and staying well. In fact, studies show that lifestyle interventions are the most effective treatment for reversing prediabetes, lowering hemoglobin A1C, decreasing high blood pressure, improving fitness, and promoting weight loss (Wing and the Look AHEAD Research Group 2010). During the prediabetes detox, you will need to exercise regularly, get plenty of sleep, manage stress effectively, take saunas or hot baths, and quit smoking if you smoke. Fortunately, the side effects are all positive: waking up well rested, having plenty of energy throughout the day, feeling happier and less stressed, experiencing fewer food cravings, and being able to better concentrate, focus, and remember.

The prediabetes detox has five lifestyle guidelines:

1. Stop smoking.

2. Exercise for five hours each week.

3. Manage stress effectively.

4. Get at least nine hours of sleep each night.

5. Take saunas, or warm Epsom salt baths, regularly.

These activities work together to support detoxification. Exercising regularly, managing stress, and getting enough sleep help keep insulin levels low, allowing your body to burn fat and mobilize toxins. Exercise also increases circulation of blood and lymphatic fluid throughout the body, increasing the removal of waste products from tissues, and along with sauna therapy, it supports pathways of elimination, allowing your body to excrete toxins that have been mobilized and detoxified by your liver.

Most of these activities should become permanent parts of your lifestyle. Sauna therapy is most important during detox, but you'll need to get regular exercise, sleep well, and manage stress for the rest of your life. This chapter covers each of these guidelines in detail.

1. Stop Smoking

There is nothing good about smoking. It's toxic for the people who do it and for the people around them who are exposed to second-hand smoke. Studies show that smoking raises fasting blood sugar levels and increases the risk for diabetes, among many other illnesses like cancer and cardiovascular disease (Rafalson et al. 2009).

Cigarettes are physically and psychologically addictive, and stopping smoking can be difficult, so seek help if you need it. Close to 90 percent of successful long-term quitters stopped smoking abruptly, and this cold turkey method has been shown to be twice as effective as nicotine replacement therapy and medications that are taken to reduce cravings (Dorana et al. 2006). Drugs carry side effects like constipation and insomnia, and nicotine replacement isn't a good choice for people with prediabetes, because studies show that long-term use can increase levels of insulin and promote insulin resistance (Eliasson, Taskinen, and Smith 1996). If you can't quit cold turkey on your own, talk to your naturopathic doctor about alternative therapies like taking botanical medicines to reduce your desire to smoke and help heal your lungs. Acupuncture and hypnosis may also be helpful.

Even if you don't smoke, being exposed to secondhand smoke can increase your risk for diabetes. Compared to nonsmokers, people exposed to secondhand smoke have higher levels of fasting blood sugar, higher hemoglobin A1C, more insulin resistance, and a higher rate of type 2 diabetes (Tweed et al. 2012). Whenever possible, avoid exposure to secondhand smoke.

2. Exercise for Five Hours Each Week

Exercise has so many benefits. It helps reverse prediabetes by reducing inflammation, lowering blood sugar, and making cells more sensitive to insulin (Thomas, Elliott, and Naughton 2006). It boosts levels of serotonin, which helps reduce food cravings. It aids detoxification by burning fat, mobilizing toxins, making you sweat, increasing air exchange, and increasing lymphatic circulation. Because lymphatic vessels have thin walls that don't effectively pump fluids through, they rely on contraction of the surrounding muscles. Without regular physical activity and muscle movement, the lymphatic system doesn't work well and garbage builds up inside the body. Taking out the garbage is an essential part of detoxification.

Exercise is also important for good overall health, for it lowers high blood pressure and triglycerides (a form of fat in the blood that increases the risk of cardiovascular disease), improves mitochondrial function and energy production, strengthens bones and muscles, releases feel-good compounds called endorphins, helps manage stress, fights premature aging (Huebschmann, Kohrt, and Regensteiner 2011), and modulates genetic expression through epigenetic mechanisms (Sanchis-Gomar et al. 2012). Exercise can also improve digestion, sleep, mood, concentration, coordination, balance, and flexibility.

Studies show that regular exercise improves fitness in people with high blood sugar by as much as 40 percent in as little as three to five months (Huebschmann, Kohrt, and Regensteiner 2011). The best forms of exercise are the ones you'll do regularly, so find activities that you enjoy. Exercising at a gym is a great option, especially when the weather is bad, when the gym is equipped with a sauna, and when it offers classes that inspire and motivate you to exercise. But gyms aren't really necessary. You can exercise on your own at home by practicing yoga, using resistance bands, jumping rope, jumping on a trampoline (which is also called rebounding and is especially good for stimulating lymphatic circulation), and doing push-ups, pull-ups, stomach crunches, and squats. You can exercise outdoors by hiking, biking, speed walking, swimming, skiing, or ice skating and get your daily dose of sunshine at the same time. You can play a partnered sport, like tennis or squash, or a team sport, like crew, basketball, volleyball, softball, or soccer. Or you can exercise recreationally by gardening or salsa dancing. If you have joint problems, choose activities with little or no impact, like swimming, aqua exercise (inside a pool), bicycling, or using an elliptical machine.

If you aren't already physically active or if you want to intensify your current routine, first talk to your doctor to make sure that it's safe for you, and discuss whether there are any activities that you should specifically avoid or attempt, based on your needs and goals. Once you get permission to exercise, consider meeting at least once with a personal trainer, who can put together an appropriate routine for you, familiarize you with exercise equipment, and make sure you're doing your exercises correctly. Personal training sessions are also a good way to get motivated and stay focused, especially if you need a structured program to make it happen.

Start with one hour of exercise five times per week. Later, once your blood sugar and insulin levels normalize, you may be able to reduce your routine to three hours each week. But for now, for detoxification, and for getting your blood sugar and insulin levels under control, you need to exercise for five hours each week.

Be sure to incorporate all three types of exercise: aerobic, strengthening, and stretching. Each one has unique benefits, and our bodies need them all. One study found that for people with high blood sugar, the combination of aerobic and strengthening exercises was far more powerful than either type of exercise alone (Church et al. 2010). Compared to people who didn't exercise and those who did only aerobic or strengthening exercises, those who did both lost more weight, and they were the only ones to lower their hemoglobin A1C levels. Another study followed more than thirty-two thousand men for eighteen years and found that those who performed at least 150 minutes of aerobic and strengthening exercises each week reduced their risk of type 2 diabetes by almost 60 percent (Grøntved et al. 2012).

Aerobic Exercise

Sometimes called *cardio,* aerobic exercise increases your heart rate and breathing rate and makes you sweat. Before and after aerobic activity, you should always warm up and cool down to allow your body's circulatory, neuromuscular, and metabolic systems to adapt to the changing levels of physical exertion. To warm up and cool down, you can do the same type of exercise but with less intensity, like biking on a flat surface before biking uphill, or you can change activities, like walking before jumping rope. Spend at least five minutes warming up and at least five minutes cooling down.

Whatever form of aerobic exercise you choose, you should incorporate *interval training,* the practice of alternating short bursts of higher intensity activity with periods of lower intensity exercise that allow muscles to recover. Changing the intensity can involve altering the speed, resistance, or incline of an activity. Research studies show that interval training increases exercise capacity (Burgomaster et al. 2005) and stimulates the body to burn more fat (Talanian et al. 2007). Interval training can be done with almost any activity.

During high-intensity intervals, you should be giving an all-out effort. You should feel a burning sensation in your muscles, and it should leave you out of breath. Before and after high-intensity intervals, exercise at moderate intensity and do not allow your heart rate to return to a resting rate. Space high-intensity intervals at least four minutes apart and allow at least two days between sessions of interval training. Start by adding one high-intensity interval of thirty seconds to your aerobic routine and gradually work your way up to three high-intensity intervals of one to four minutes each, three times per week.

Checking your heart rate is a good idea. I don't want you to get hung up on numbers and measurements, but you should be sure that you're exercising enough. Some people like to wear heart-rate monitors, but it's not really necessary. A regular watch and some simple math will work just fine. Use your fingertips to find the pulse inside your opposite wrist or on the side of your neck just below your jaw, count the beats for ten seconds, and multiply by six.

Your maximum heart rate (MHR) is equal to 220 minus your age in years. Your target heart rate (THR) for moderate-intensity exercise is between 50 and 70 percent of your maximum heart rate. Your THR for high-intensity exercise is between 70 and 85 percent of your MHR.

To calculate your target heart rates, subtract your age from 220. In three different equations, multiply this number by 0.5, by 0.7, and by 0.85 to find your THR ranges for 50, 70, and 85 percent of your maximum heart rate. If you divide these numbers by six, you'll find the number of heartbeats you should have per ten seconds.

For example, a fifty-year-old woman has a maximum heart rate of 170 beats per minute. Her target heart rate for moderate-intensity exercise is between 85 beats per minute (50 percent MHR) and 119 beats per minute (70 percent MHR), or between 14 and 20 beats per ten seconds. Her target heart rate for high-intensity exercise is between 119 beats per minute (70 percent MHR) and 144 beats per minute (85 percent MHR), or between 20 and 24 beats per ten seconds.

Realize that these numbers are good guidelines, but they're only approximations. Ultimately, how you feel is more important than how fast your heart is beating. If you ever experience chest pain or feel light-headed or short of breath, stop exercising, rest, and make an appointment to discuss it with your doctor. If you are taking certain heart medications like beta blockers, these equations don't apply to you. Before exercising, ask your doctor to recommend the THRs most appropriate for you.

Strengthening Exercise

Strengthening exercise can also be called *resistance* exercise or *weight-bearing* exercise. This form of exertion stimulates the growth of muscle cells and bone cells, which makes your skeleton stronger. Strengthening exercise also improves the sensitivity of insulin receptors on cells, allowing them to take up glucose from the blood more efficiently, reduces hemoglobin A1C, and significantly reduces the risk of developing type 2 diabetes. One study showed that in as little as ten weeks, resistance training increased lean body mass by more than three pounds, reduced fat mass by nearly four pounds, and increased resting metabolic rate by 7 percent (Westcott 2012). The effects of exercise on insulin receptors are almost immediate and can last for days.

In addition to lifting weights or using resistance machines, resistance bands, or kettlebells, strengthening exercises include playing basketball or volleyball, speed walking, doing push-ups and lunges, rebounding, and practicing pilates and some forms of yoga.

You should spend at least an hour each week doing strengthening exercises and divide the time into multiple sessions: thirty minutes two times per week, twenty minutes three times per week, or fifteen minutes four times per week. Avoid exercising the same muscles on consecutive days, for they require a day of rest and repair between sessions. If you plan to do separate aerobic and strengthening exercises during the same workout, do the strength training first. Performing strengthening exercise before aerobic exercise can increase the amount of fat you burn (Goto et al. 2007). If you're working with resistance machines or free weights, perform at least one exercise for each muscle group twice each week. You can focus on all areas during one session, or you can split them up, alternating exercises for your upper body (arms, chest, abdomen) one day with exercises for your lower body (legs and back) another day.

For each exercise, you should do three sets of ten repetitions with little or no rest between sets. The weight should be heavy enough to fatigue your muscles and make finishing the last repetition difficult but attainable. After you've finished all three sets of one exercise, rest for one minute before you move on to the next exercise.

To prevent unnecessary stress on the body that could raise cortisol levels (along with blood sugar and insulin levels), don't engage in strength training for more than forty-five minutes at a time and don't attempt to lift weights that are too heavy for you. If you're using heavy free weights, you should work with a spotter, either a personal trainer or a workout partner strong enough to lift the weights you're using.

Stretching Exercise

Stretching exercises are important for preventing and easing muscle tension and maintaining flexible and healthy joints. To avoid

115

the risk of strain and injury, stretch your muscles only after you've warmed up. You can also stretch during your workout if your muscles feel tense, tight, or sore. Here are some basic stretching guidelines:

- Always stretch at the end of your workout, even if you stretched earlier in your routine.

- Stretch all of your muscle groups: arms, chest, abdomen, back, and legs.

- Ease into and out of stretches slowly.

- Hold each position for fifteen seconds or more.

- Never bounce while you stretch.

- Do not exceed the comfortable range of motion. Stretching should never be painful.

If you need specific ideas for stretching exercises, visit www .prediabetesdetox.com.

Basic Exercise Guidelines

During the prediabetes detox, you should spend a total of five hours each week doing a combination of aerobic and strengthening exercises. Interval training will add intense bursts of activity, but otherwise exercise should be of moderate intensity. Too much high-intensity exercise can actually raise cortisol levels and increase the risk of insulin resistance.

As you plan your exercise routine, keep in mind that longer periods of aerobic exercise are better for burning fat. During the first twenty minutes or so of exercise, muscles use sugar stored as glycogen for energy. Once glycogen reserves have been depleted, muscles start burning fat for energy. To maximize the burning of fat and the mobilization of toxins, plan to spend at least thirty to forty-five minutes doing aerobic exercise whenever possible. Limit your workouts to one hour (aerobic and strengthening exercises combined) to prevent raising cortisol levels.

Warming up, cooling down, and stretching must also be done in addition to the five hours of aerobic and strengthening exercises. For examples of two weekly exercise regimens, one that you can do in a gym and one that you can do without a gym, visit www.prediabetes-detox.com. In addition to warming up and cooling down, drink plenty of water before and after you exercise. Skip the sports beverages and drink pure, unsweetened coconut water instead, or consume foods high in electrolytes at your next meal to replenish those lost during your workout. Foods high in elecrolytes include celery, broccoli, artichokes, mustard greens, spinach, sardines, haddock, and wild Alaskan salmon.

As important as it is to exercise, it's equally important to avoid being sedentary. Even if you work out every day, sitting for long periods of time can contribute to the same disease processes as not exercising at all (Craft et al. 2012). Whenever you're seated, get up at least once an hour to move around for at least a minute. Do some jumping jacks, take a short stroll, climb some stairs, or do some simple range-of-motion exercises for your neck, arms, hips, and legs to increase circulation. If you need a reminder, set an alarm on your computer, phone, or watch.

3. Manage Stress Effectively

A certain amount of stress is unavoidable. In small doses it can be good for us, but in big doses it can be dangerous. During times of physical and psychological stress, our adrenal glands (a pair of small organs that sit on top of the kidneys) increase their production of the stress hormone cortisol. As part of an inherent survival instinct, cortisol prepares the body for fight-or-flight action by raising alertness, increasing heart rate and blood pressure, and boosting levels of blood sugar and insulin. Cortisol also increases our appetite for sweets and starches because these foods raise blood sugar levels quickly, providing our muscles with immediate fuel.

When we're continuously exposed to stress, whether physical or mental, real or imagined, levels of cortisol are continuously elevated. This triggers inflammation, prompts the body to accumulate fat, interferes with detoxification, increases the risk of developing diabetes, and alters gene expression through epigenetic mechanisms (Godfrey, Inskip, and Hanson 2011). High cortisol levels also deplete serotonin, a neurotransmitter (or chemical messenger in the brain) that helps regulate appetite and mood. When levels of serotonin are low, we crave sweet and starchy foods, and we're more likely to binge or overeat. Low levels of serotonin can also cause depression or anxiety, which makes coping with stress even more challenging.

When levels of cortisol are low, the body can regulate blood sugar and insulin more effectively, as long as you avoid fast carbs. One of the best ways to keep cortisol levels low is to find activities that lower your stress level. Exercise is a good one, but other options are also effective, especially those that promote relaxation like yoga, breathing exercises, meditation, guided imagery, progressive muscle relaxation, qigong, massage, or simply spending time in nature. Relaxation is a skill, so if it doesn't come naturally to you, you can learn to do it well. As with any skill, relaxation requires practice, focus, and concentration. The more you do it, the easier it will be. Pick the activity or activities that feel right to you, and practice them daily or whenever the need arises.

Also understand that your thoughts and feelings affect your stress levels. While you can't control what happens to you, you can control how you react to what happens to you. Painful emotions like anger, fear, grief, and sadness certainly have their place in our lives, but we must also learn to let them go.

Yoga

Yoga has big benefits for people with prediabetes. Studies show that regular practice can lower levels of blood sugar and insulin, promote weight loss, and boost levels of glutathione (Hegde et al. 2011). It can also improve insulin sensitivity, lower cortisol levels, and reduce inflammation (Innes and Vincent 2007).

There are several different styles of yoga:

- *Hatha* yoga is gentle, slow paced, and focused on breathing and meditation.

- *Vinyasa* yoga combines breathing exercises with basic physical poses.

- *Ashtanga* yoga combines breathing exercises with an intense, fast-paced series of poses.

- *Iyengar* yoga focuses on body alignment. It uses standing poses and props like blocks to strengthen the body.

- *Bikram* yoga is a series of twenty-six poses practiced at a temperature of 95 to 100°F.

- *Hot* yoga is similar to Bikram yoga.

Some forms of yoga can be aerobic if they raise your heart rate and breathing rate and they make you sweat, and they can be strengthening if you're doing poses that use your body weight to place force on your bones. Other forms of yoga are good for stretching. If you're interested in yoga, look for a class in your community. If you can't find personal instruction, look for a DVD that you like.

Basic Breathing Exercises

Slow and steady breathing helps our bodies relax by stimulating the vagus nerve, which connects our hearts and lungs to our brains. It doesn't take a lot of time to see results, and it can be done anywhere. There are lots of good breathing exercises. Here is just one example:

1. Position yourself comfortably so that your spine is straight.

2. Inhale deeply through your nose for a count of four.

3. Hold your breath for a count of six.

4. Exhale fully, deflating your abdomen, for a count of eight.

5. Repeat.

Perform this exercise for several minutes to relax during times of stress, or use it to induce sleep at bedtime.

Meditation

Meditation is a self-directed practice for relaxing the body and calming the mind. It's been shown to boost levels of serotonin, reduce levels of cortisol, increase levels of melatonin, regulate metabolism, and improve sleep (Nagendra, Maruthai, and Kutty1 2012).

There are several different techniques. *Transcendental* meditation focuses on a mantra (a chosen sound, word, or phrase) and attempts to transcend daily concerns. *Mindfulness* meditation focuses on breathing and self-awareness and attempts to improve the way we react to stress. One form of mindfulness meditation called *integrative body–mind training* (IBMT), adapted from traditional Chinese medicine, focuses on achieving a state of restful alertness under the active guidance of a coach. IBMT was found to induce positive structural changes in the brain associated with an improved response to stress after only eleven hours of practice (Tang 2011). For an example of a simple meditation exercise and a link to more information about IBMT, visit www.prediabetesdetox.com.

Guided Imagery

During guided imagery, you can guide yourself through a peaceful and relaxing situation, or someone else can guide you, either a live person or a recording. Before you start, find a quiet and comfortable place. Then imagine yourself inside a scene that makes you happy, perhaps lying in a field of wildflowers or walking on a beach. With guided imagery, you use your senses to fully appreciate the details of the scene. Can you smell the perfume of the flowers or the saltiness of the ocean? Is the sunshine warm on your skin or the water cool on your feet? You can spend as much time as you like in this scene and return whenever you want, even if you just have a minute or two in the middle of a busy day.

Progressive Muscle Relaxation

Progressive muscle relaxation helps relax the body by reducing tension in major muscle groups. To do this exercise, find a quiet place where you will be undisturbed. If you are not trying to induce sleep, do it in a seated position. Dim the lighting. Close your eyes. Concentrate on deep, slow breathing. Tense and relax each of the major muscle groups slowly and in sequence, starting with your head and scalp, and moving down to your face, neck, shoulders, upper arms, lower arms, hands and fingers, chest, abdomen, upper and lower back, hips, thighs, calves, feet, and toes. Feel a sensation of lightness as tension is released. Remain relaxed as long as you wish. Then slowly open your eyes, emerging calm and refreshed (unless you are using this technique to induce sleep).

Qigong

Qigong means "movement of energy." It is a popular Chinese practice that combines mental concentration, breathing exercises, and simple physical movements to increase the flow of energy in the body. According to Chinese medicine philosophy, illness results from congestion and stagnation, and anything that creates movement, relieves congestion, and removes stagnation will be beneficial to your health. When energy (or *qi*) flows freely and evenly through the body, healing can take place. Qigong is used to manage stress, relieve muscle tension, increase circulation, and improve sleep. Practice it in the morning to help you wake up and greet the new day, in the middle of a busy day to help you regain your focus and concentration for tasks at hand, or after a long day to help you unwind and relax. For an example of a simple qigong exercise, visit www.prediabetesdetox.com.

Massage

Getting a massage is a good way to relax and manage stress. It also boosts serotonin and supports detoxification by increasing lymphatic circulation. Specific massage techniques exist that are designed to increase the flow of lymphatic fluid, but all forms of massage will do this to some degree.

Forest Bathing

Forest bathing means being surrounded by a forest environment. It may not seem like therapy, but forest bathing has been shown to reduce stress and lower blood sugar levels. One Japanese study followed eighty-seven adults diagnosed with type 2 diabetes for six years (Ohtsuka, Yabunaka, and Takayama 1998). During this time, participants walked in a forest for three or six kilometers (1.9 or 3.7 miles), depending on their physical ability, on nine different occasions. At the end of the study, researchers found that they had lower blood sugar, improved insulin sensitivity, and decreased levels of hemoglobin A1C. This wasn't a controlled study, and any form of exercise practiced regularly can help improve blood sugar regulation in people with diabetes. But given the frequency of the walks (only nine times in six years) and the fact that blood sugar levels were significantly decreased but not significantly different between those who walked the long distance and those who walked the short distance, researchers concluded that factors other than exercise contributed to the positive long-term effects.

In Japan, forest bathing (or *shinrin-yoku*) has had such positive effects that some companies include it in employee health care benefits and wellness programs, and free checkups are even available inside Japanese forests. Researchers believe that the health benefits are related to compounds called *phytoncides* in the forest air. Phytoncides are essential oils released by trees and plants to defend themselves against insects, animals, and decomposition.

If you can, spend time outside every week, preferably in a natural environment full of plants and trees. Forests are ideal, but parks are good alternatives.

4. Get at Least Nine Hours of Sleep Each Night

Like exercise and stress management, getting good sleep is just as important for reversing prediabetes as it is for detoxification. Our circadian rhythms are dictated by light-and-dark cycles, and they help to regulate blood sugar and insulin levels. Every one of our cells has an internal clock that responds to changes in daylight. Special proteins called *cryptochromes* in our skin cells are sensitive to light's blue spectrum, so whenever we're bathed in light, our bodies get the message to wake up. Light exposure causes cortisol levels to go up, along with blood sugar and insulin levels. Light also causes levels of melatonin, a hormone that helps us sleep, to go down.

When we get lots of sleep, we increase the amount of time we spend in darkness and decrease the amount of time we're exposed to light. Longer nights and shorter days mean that our bodies make more melatonin and less cortisol, which can cause blood sugar and insulin levels to go down. This pattern of light-and-dark cycles mimics winter, when food is naturally less abundant, our appetite is naturally suppressed, and our bodies burn fat for fuel.

When we don't get enough sleep, we decrease the amount of time we spend in darkness and increase the amount of time we're exposed to light. Shorter nights and longer days mean that we make less melatonin and more cortisol, which can cause blood sugar and insulin levels to go up. This pattern of light-and-dark cycles mimics summer, when food is naturally more abundant and we naturally crave foods we can store as fat, in anticipation for the upcoming winter when food may be scarce.

In our modern world full of artificial light, it's always summer inside our bodies. We've put an end to seasonal variations, now that days are always long, nights are always short, and the sugar and starches we crave are available year-round. Short sleep cycles raise blood sugar levels, cause cells to lose sensitivity to insulin, and increase the risk for diabetes (Knutson and Van Cauter 2008). Lack of sleep also causes levels of leptin, a hormone that reduces appetite, to go down, and levels of ghrelin, a hormone that makes you hungry, to go up. In one study of healthy men without preexisting blood sugar imbalances, being deprived of just two hours sleep caused them to crave sugar and eat more of it (Van Cauter et al. 2007). The effects are even more dramatic in people with prediabetes.

You need to get at least nine hours of sleep per night during detoxification. Research shows that when we sleep seven hours or less overnight, epigenetic changes prompt our bodies to store fat, but when we sleep nine hours or more, epigenetic influences on body weight are suppressed (Watson et al. 2012). Nine hours is a lot of sleep, but it's essential for keeping blood sugar and insulin levels low. Because sleep boosts serotonin, it also fights food cravings and it may improve your mood as well. If you're sleep deprived, you will always feel hungry and crave carbohydrates, you won't be able to detoxify effectively, and you'll have a hard time reversing prediabetes.

Unless you already sleep nine hours each night, you'll need to make more time for sleeping. Choose an earlier bedtime over a later wake time to maximize deep sleep, which usually occurs before early morning hours. Once you've determined your wake time, count backward nine hours to determine your bedtime. If you can, wake up at the same time each morning and go to bed at the same time each night, even on your days off. Try to eat your meals and exercise at the same times each day too. Keeping a regular schedule and being consistent supports a healthy circadian rhythm, which promotes good sleep, blood sugar control, and overall well-being.

If you have problems falling asleep or staying asleep, resist the urge to get up, and do not turn on the light. Avoid electronic gadgets at night, as they can lower levels of melatonin, raise levels of cortisol, and cause problems with falling asleep, staying asleep, and controlling blood sugar. It's common for people to want to get up and be productive if they can't sleep, and while it's not ideal to associate your bed with insomnia and anxiety, the bottom line is that if you get up and stimulate your mind, even if you don't turn on the lights, your cortisol levels will go up, making it unlikely that you'll fall asleep later, and even if you do, you won't get the same benefits. Instead, I recommend practicing breathing exercises, meditation, guided imagery, progressive muscle relaxation, or self-hypnosis to calm your mind and slow brain activity.

Follow these tips to maximize your sleep:

- Avoid caffeine and alcohol, especially in the evening. Alcohol acts as a central nervous system depressant and may cause you to fall asleep, but it also interferes with deep-sleep mechanisms, causes awakenings during the night, and reduces sleep quality.

- Exercise in the morning if you can. Avoid exercising after dinner and after 8:00 p.m.

- Finish eating at least three hours before you go to bed.

- Limit liquids in the evening if you wake up to urinate during the night.

- After dark and especially after 9:00 p.m., keep your lights as dim as possible. Studies show that exposure to regular room light can shorten melatonin secretion by ninety minutes in 99 percent of people (Gooley et al. 2011).

- Avoid watching TV, playing video games, talking on your cell phone, and using computers, laptops, tablets, and all other electronic devices after 9:00 p.m. and at least one hour before bed. (If you want to read before bed, opt for a real book over an electronic book.) On occasions when you must use electronic devices, keep them as far away from your head as possible. Also consider wearing glasses with amber, rose, or orange lenses to block blue light. Research has shown that wearing amber-colored glasses before bed can simulate darkness and maximize melatonin levels (Phelps 2008).

- Set aside a half hour or more to relax and unwind before bed.

- Use your bedroom for sleep and sex only. And don't neglect the sex. Pleasurable sexual activity, whether alone or with a partner, is good for you. It balances hormones and normalizes neurotransmitters that help regulate fat metabolism. Good sex also helps relieve stress, lower high blood pressure, boost immunity, improve sleep, reduce pain, and bolster self-esteem.

- Make sure your sleeping environment is quiet, comfortable, and cool. Use nontoxic, good-quality bed linens, pillows, and mattress (organic cotton is a good choice). Maintain an overnight temperature in your bedroom between 62°F (in the winter) and 68°F (in the summer).

- Do not use wireless devices as alarm clocks, and remove as many electronic devices from your bedroom as you can. Ideally, you'll only need lamps with dim lighting and a battery-powered alarm clock that doesn't glow in the dark. If you can, use one that wakes you with gradual light or gentle sounds rather than loud or startling noises. If you must use a clock that emits light at night, pick one that glows red instead of blue. And if you can't live without a phone in your bedroom, use a corded landline instead of a cellular or cordless phone.

- If you have a wireless router in your home, keep it as far away from your bedroom as possible.

- Don't sleep with kids or pets.

- If you have indoor allergies, consider installing a high-efficiency particulate air (HEPA) filter system to remove dust and other particulates from the air in your sleeping environment. Also use a vacuum equipped with a HEPA filter regularly.

- Sleep in complete darkness. Wearing an eye mask isn't enough. Get black-out curtains if any artificial light shines through your windows at night. (If none shines through, leave your curtains open to allow the morning sunshine to wake you up naturally.) If you must use night-lights, find ones that glow amber, rose, or orange instead of white or blue.

- Get up as close to sunrise as possible and spend ten to twenty minutes outside everyday, as early as possible. If you can, go barefoot or wear leather-soled shoes on grass, sand, dirt, or gravel surfaces. Connecting your body to the earth and exposing your skin to early morning sunshine resets your circadian rhythm, helps regulate blood sugar and fat metabolism, improves sleep patterns, normalizes stress hormones, and increases the natural production of serotonin and endorphins, the opiate-like compounds that make us happy and calm (Mead 2008).

Avoid intense or excessive sun exposure and don't leave your skin exposed long enough to develop a sunburn.

Vitamin G

Earthing or *grounding*, also known as "vitamin G," simply means maintaining physical contact with the earth. Our planet's surface has an abundance of negatively charged free electrons able to neutralize positively charged free radicals inside our bodies. Maintaining regular contact with the earth can reduce inflammation and improve blood sugar control in people with diabetes (Sokal and Sokal 2011).

Ironically, earthing can now be done artificially with electron transfer technology. A wide range of conductive appliances are available, including mattresses, bedsheets, mats, body bands, shoes, and electrode patches you stick on your skin. These devices may interfere with blood-thinning medications, and people who use them may experience adverse effects like muscle cramps, tingling sensations, and flu-like symptoms.

The best way to connect to the earth is by going barefoot on surfaces that conduct electrons: grass, sand, dirt, gravel, concrete surfaces, or natural water sources. Wet surfaces conduct electrons even better than dry surfaces, so strolling on the beach or walking in dew-covered grass is even better. If you can't be barefoot, the next best thing is to wear leather-soled shoes, which conduct some electrons. Rubber- and plastic-soled shoes don't conduct electrons at all.

5. Take Saunas or Warm Epsom Salt Baths Regularly

Sauna therapy uses dry heat to warm the body and stimulate elimination of toxins through sweat. A study of rescue workers from the 9/11 World Trade Center attack demonstrated that sauna therapy can effectively reduce levels of environmental toxins in the blood, including dioxins and PCBs (Dahlgren et al. 2007). The rescue workers followed the Hubbard protocol, a daily regimen of physical exercise followed by two and a half hours inside a sauna of 140 to 180°F (allowing for short breaks as needed) and supplementation of vitamins and minerals. After sauna therapy, dioxin levels were undetectable, PCB levels had dropped by 65 percent, and all rescue workers reported a reversal of their symptoms.

Traditional saunas are one good option and far-infrared saunas are another. While traditional saunas heat the room, far-infrared saunas heat the body directly using radiant heat and invisible light waves to penetrate tissues. Far-infrared sauna therapy has been studied specifically in people with high blood sugar, and researchers found that taking a twenty-minute far-infrared sauna three times per week for three months improved fatigue, depression, pain, and overall quality of life for people with type 2 diabetes (Beever 2010). Far-infrared saunas can be more comfortable than traditional saunas because air temperatures are cooler, usually between 90 and 115°F. You probably won't feel overheated inside a far-infrared sauna, but because its effects are more intense than those of a traditional sauna, you should still limit your exposure. If you're using a far-infrared sauna, do one twenty-minute session, followed by a cold shower of thirty seconds or more, five to seven times per week.

If you're using a traditional sauna, begin with one fifteen-minute session, followed by a cold shower of thirty seconds or more. If you tolerate the first session well, increase the number of sessions during subsequent treatments until you build up to four fifteen-minute sessions per treatment, each followed by a cold shower. Perform five to seven treatments each week.

Make sure the sauna you're using is made of natural wood and nontoxic materials. There shouldn't be any parts made of plastic, chemical-treated wood, or other materials that would release toxins into the air. It's still a good idea to leave the door slightly ajar for ventilation.

To increase sweating during the sauna, you can drink ginger tea or take five hundred milligrams of ginger in supplement form about thirty minutes beforehand. To stay hydrated during the sauna, drink one cup (eight ounces) of filtered water, ginger tea, or coconut water before and after each session, or while you're inside the sauna. In hotter saunas you may feel more comfortable with a cold, wet towel wrapped around your head and/or a cool, wet washcloth on your forehead. If at any time inside the sauna you feel dizzy, nauseous, or overheated, you should leave, drink some water, take a cold shower, and rest until you feel well again.

After each sauna treatment, there are three things you should do:

1. Take a shower or bath and wash your body well to remove any toxins that were secreted from your skin. (Find my recipe for an easy homemade sea salt scrub at www.prediabetes detox.com.)

2. Rest for at least twenty minutes.

3. Consume plenty of foods rich in electrolytes at your next meal to replace the ones you sweated out.

Traditional and infrared sauna therapy is usually safe and well tolerated for most people. It has been contraindicated for people with high blood pressure or heart disease, but studies show that people with these conditions actually benefit from sauna therapy (Crinnion 2011). Use of all saunas should be avoided during early pregnancy, but so should detoxification.

Epsom Salt Baths

Sauna therapy is best, but if you don't have access to a sauna, a warm bath with Epsom salts (magnesium sulfate) is the next best thing. It hasn't been studied in regard to detoxification, but like a sauna, it will raise your body temperature and make you sweat. You should be able to find Epsom salts at any drugstore.

Add two cups of Epsom salts to a warm bath and relax for twenty to thirty minutes. If desired, add five to ten drops of pure essential oil (like lavender, which promotes relaxation) after you fill the tub. (The essential oils will evaporate much more quickly if you add them to hot running water.) End your bath with a cold shower of thirty seconds or more.

Like sauna therapy, Epsom salt baths can make you sleepy, so rest afterward or consider taking these baths just before bed. They can also be dehydrating, so drink one cup (eight ounces) of water or ginger tea before your bath and again afterward, and consume plenty of electrolytes at your next meal.

A Healthy Lifestyle

If you haven't already, now is the time to make a firm commitment to a healthy lifestyle. Make time to exercise regularly, get plenty of sleep, spend time relaxing, and at least for the time being, take saunas or hot baths. Put these activities at the top of your priority list and find a way to make them happen.

chapter 6

Detoxification for Your Home

The United States makes twenty-seven trillion pounds of chemicals each year, which amounts to almost seventy-four billion pounds per day. Unlike laws in Europe that require new chemicals to be proven safe before they are put on the market, laws in the United States allow chemicals to be used until they are proven unsafe. There are almost eighty thousand different chemicals used in the United States, but only a few hundred of them have ever been tested for safety (Reuben 2010). The President's Cancer Panel reported that the majority of chemicals in our environment are unstudied or understudied and largely unregulated (Reuben 2010), and the Environmental Protection Agency admits that "most Americans would assume that basic toxicity testing is available and that all chemicals in commerce today are safe," but "this is not a prudent assumption" (EPA 2008).

According to the EPA (2008), a full set of basic safety information is available for only 7 percent of the high volume chemicals manufactured in the United States, nearly half of the chemicals have never been tested at all, and only five have ever been restricted. These chemicals don't occur in isolation, and while we have little information about individual chemicals, we have even less about chemicals in combination. It would be practically impossible to study all of the interactions between tens of thousands of toxins, but that's the way that we're exposed to them. At any given time, dozens or even hundreds of harmful substances surround us. Chemicals from carpeting, paint, furniture, electronic devices, and air fresheners escape as gas particles into the air we breathe. Other toxins from fabrics, personal products, household cleaners, and electromagnetic radiation come into direct contact with our bodies and are readily absorbed through our skin.

Toxins begin to build up inside our bodies before we're even born. According to research studies, already at birth, babies' bodies contain mercury, multiple pesticides, more than a dozen different flame retardants, and air pollutants from fossil fuels, plastic production, and coal-fired power plants. The Environmental Working Group, in partnership with laboratories around the world, has found 232 different chemicals in the cord blood of newborn infants and 493 different chemicals in people of all ages (EWG 2009b).

We'll never be able to completely escape environmental toxins, but we can take precautions to minimize our exposure. Your home is a good place to start, for you spend a lot of your time there, and unlike other environments, it's largely under your control. This chapter will focus on the environmental toxins found outside of foods that have been linked to an increased risk of diabetes.

Environmental Toxins

Some environmental toxins associated with prediabetes are impossible to avoid, like those found in air pollution, but others we can take reasonable measures to evade. In addition to those listed in chapter 2, they include parabens, flame retardants, volatile organic compounds, and electromagnetic radiation.

Parabens

Parabens are a family of chemicals that includes methylparaben, propylparaben, and butylparaben. Because parabens act as preservatives, they're used by manufacturers to extend shelf life. They're found in prescription drugs, food additives, and personal products like shampoo, lotion, deodorant, and cosmetics. According to the

FDA, parabens are the most widely used preservatives in cosmetics, and they're often used in combination with other preservatives. Studies show that parabens act as endocrine disruptors and interfere with insulin production (Boberg et al. 2008).

Volatile Organic Compounds

Volatile organic compounds are chemicals used in manufacturing that escape from products in the form of gases. They're found in paint, carpet, building materials, glues, adhesives, permanent markers, office equipment such as copiers and printers, household cleaners, pesticides, auto exhaust, and fragranced products like air fresheners and scented candles. According to the EPA, VOCs are up to ten times more concentrated in indoor air than in outdoor air (EPA 2012a), and studies show that they promote high blood sugar and insulin resistance (Hong et al. 2009).

Flame Retardants

Brominated flame retardants (BFRs) are added to furniture, electronic equipment like computers and televisions, mattresses, and clothing like children's sleepwear. Because BFRs don't break down very easily, they've become persistent and widespread in the environment. Like parabens, BFRs act as endocrine disruptors, and studies have linked them to obesity and type 2 diabetes (Casals-Casas and Desvergne 2011).

Electromagnetic Radiation

Studies show that electromagnetic radiation (EMR) produced by electronic devices and Wi-Fi technology can raise blood sugar levels (Havas 2008), alter blood sugar metabolism in the tissues it penetrates (Volkow et al. 2011), deplete glutathione (Keyse and Tyrrell 1987), and disrupt sleep (Akerstedt et al. 1999). In fact, exposure to even commonly occurring low-frequency electromagnetic fields significantly reduces both the quality and quantity of sleep (Akerstedt et al. 1999). Less sleep means higher levels of blood sugar and insulin and an increased risk of developing diabetes (see chapter 5).

Detoxing Your Home

Whether we realize it or not, harmful chemicals linked to prediabetes lurk inside our homes. Follow these twelve tips to minimize your exposure or to avoid them completely.

1. Take Off Your Shoes

One of the easiest ways to prevent outdoor toxins from becoming indoor toxins is to leave your shoes at the door. Politely insist that everyone else do so too.

2. Open the Windows

According to the EPA, indoor air is "more seriously polluted than the outdoor air in even the largest and most industrialized cities" (EPA 2012c). To help exchange and circulate air inside your home, open your windows as often as you can. If your home has a mechanical ventilation system, use it regularly and keep it in good working order. If you have a gas stove, be sure to turn on the exhaust fan every time you use it to reduce concentrations of nitrogen dioxide, a product of combustion released as a toxic gas with potent oxidizing abilities.

3. Dust Regularly

Toxic chemicals attach themselves to household dust particles. As part of the Cape Cod Breast Cancer and Environment Study, researchers analyzed dust from 120 homes (Rudel et al. 2003). They found sixty-six different chemicals, including phthalates, flame retardants, dioxins, and twenty-seven different pesticides including dichlorodiphenyltrichloroethane (DDT). DDT has been banned in the United States for the past forty years, but it persists in the environment and was detected in 65 percent of homes (Rudel et al. 2003).

Cape Cod dust may be more or less toxic than the dust in your home, but it's still a good idea to remove dust regularly. Avoid using dusters that simply move dust around and redistribute it in the air. Instead, use a clean, damp, washable cloth to pick up dust and remove it completely. If you have indoor allergies or chemical sensitivities, you should consider installing HEPA filters and using vacuums fitted with the same.

4. Use Cleaner Cleaners

Replace chemical cleaners with white vinegar, baking soda, and essential oils. Vinegar cleans by dissolving surface residue, and baking soda acts as an abrasive agent to remove it. Essential oils disinfect because they are naturally antibacterial, and tea tree essential oil is especially effective at removing mold and mildew. Only use pure essential oils, and avoid synthetic, fragranced, and perfume or perfumed oils. Follow these tips to keep your home naturally clean:

- Clean stoves, appliances, sinks, toilets, tubs, and counters (as long as they're not made from natural stone) with Dr. Sarah's Cleaner Cleaner, a nontoxic, all-purpose cleaner (see box), or a paste made by mixing baking soda with a few drops of water or white vinegar. Baking soda paste can also remove stains from glass, ceramic, stainless steel, and silver surfaces.

- Wash natural stone countertops (marble, limestone, calcite, dolomite), dirty dishes, and delicate surfaces with liquid castile soap, made from oils like olive, coconut, hemp, and jojoba. They're gentle and nontoxic, and they don't leave a soapy residue. Do not use vinegar on natural stone surfaces, because it dissolves calcium-based stone.

- Use white vinegar to polish mirrors and windows.

- Wash uncarpeted floors with a steam mop, which uses only water and steam to clean. Alternatively, a regular mop and a solution of white vinegar and warm water can be used to clean uncarpeted floors as long as they are not made of natural stone or unfinished wood.

- To polish wooden furniture, apply olive oil to a soft cloth, rub briskly, and allow it to air dry. Do not use vinegar on wooden surfaces.

- To unclog drains, first pour a quarter cup of baking soda down the drain, and then pour in one cup of white vinegar. Wait for the foaming to subside and flush with plenty of boiling water. Don't forget to make use of drain snakes and plungers.

Dr. Sarah's Cleaner Cleaner

Use this nontoxic, all-purpose cleaner on counters, sinks, stove tops, appliances, and tiles. Do not use it on wooden, delicate, or natural stone surfaces. It smells like vinegar when it's wet, but the odor evaporates as soon as it dries.

- one cup of white vinegar
- five drops of tea tree essential oil
- five drops pure lavender or orange essential oil (avoid synthetic and perfume oils)
- one half cup of water (optional).

1. Add the ingredients to a clean glass spray bottle, close it tightly, and shake it up to mix everything together.

2. Label the bottle with the ingredients and date.

3. Before using, shake the bottle gently to redistribute the essential oils. Spray the solution on dirty surfaces, and wipe it off with a clean wet sponge. For tougher cleaning jobs, omit the water and leave the solution a few minutes before wiping off.

5. Avoid Fragrances

Manufacturers are not required to disclose additives regarded as "fragrance," and a single fragrance can contain several hundred ingredients. Remember that "unscented" doesn't necessarily mean fragrance-free, because chemicals may have been added to cover up odors.

Get rid of air fresheners, scented candles, and all fragranced household products, and, if need be, use pure essential oil diffusers instead. You can use a drop or two of pure lavender essential oil instead of perfume; it's safe to use topically, unlike other essential oils that are too caustic to be applied directly to skin.

In the laundry room, replace fragranced liquid fabric softener with a half cup of white vinegar (mixed with five drops of pure lavender or jasmine essential oil if you wish to scent your clothes), and replace fragranced dryer sheets with organic wool dryer balls.

Lavender Essential Oil

The pure essential oil of lavender can be used as a medicine, either topically on the skin's surface or internally (inside special capsules that you swallow). It should only be taken internally under the direction of a doctor. And boys should avoid all forms of it before they enter puberty, as at least one case report has indicated that it may disrupt hormone signaling in prepubescent males.

Pure lavender essential oil is generally safe for topical use, but because it is so concentrated, it should be used only in very small amounts. It's usually well tolerated, but it can cause skin reactions in people who are sensitive to it, which is true of any essential oil or plant extract. If you have allergies or sensitive skin, you can try a small amount on a small area of your skin (like the inside of your arm) and observe any reactions for forty-eight hours. If there is no irritation, you are not sensitive to lavender essential oil, and you should feel free to apply it topically in small amounts.

6. Research Your Personal Products

More than ten thousand different ingredients are used to make personal care products, and nearly 90 percent have not been evaluated for safety (EWG 2011). Learn what you're putting on your skin with the cosmetics safety database from the Environmental Working Group (find the link at www.prediabetesdetox.com). You can search by product, ingredient, or manufacturer to read toxicity information and safety reviews on items like soap, shampoo, toothpaste, deodorant, lotion, makeup, hair-styling products, nail polish, contact lens cleaner, bubble bath, sunscreen, and baby products.

I recommend rounding up all of the personal products in your home, throwing away the ones you don't use, and using the database to evaluate the ones you do. If their safety rating causes concern, use the same database to find safer alternatives.

Also consider using natural items in your personal care routine. Vinegar, yogurt, honey, almond oil, coconut oil, sea salt, oats, aloe vera, shea butter, and essential oils can all act as natural cosmetic aids. Our skin is naturally acidic, which helps it resist the growth of harmful bacteria. Soap is naturally alkaline and can reduce the natural acidity of skin. A solution of half vinegar and half water is a natural alternative to store-bought soaps and an especially good choice for people with dry skin. Vinegar removes oils and restores skin's natural pH without causing dryness. And when vinegar dries, it leaves no odor behind. You can also use the same solution as a hair rinse, to remove alkaline residues from shampoos and hair products. Rinsing hair with vinegar makes it smooth and shiny.

Yogurt and honey can condition and moisturize skin, individually or mixed together and applied just like any store-bought face mask. Yogurt also has astringent properties, causing it to constrict pores, and it supports the protective bacteria that live on the surface of your skin. Pure almond oil or coconut oil can be used to remove makeup and to moisturize skin. Coarse sea salt mixed with almond or coconut oil makes a great exfoliating and moisturizing body scrub, while finely ground oats can be mixed with pure aloe vera gel to exfoliate delicate facial skin. As an alternative to store-bought moisturizers and lotions, I make my own all-purpose salve with shea butter, almond oil, and pure essential oils. You can find this recipe and others at www.prediabetesdetox.com.

If you are allergic or sensitive to certain foods when you eat them, avoid putting them on your skin.

7. Avoid Dry-Cleaned Clothes

A volatile organic compound called tetrachloroethylene, commonly referred to as *perc*, is the most widely used solvent in the dry-cleaning industry, and it's terribly toxic. Avoid perc exposure by avoiding dry-cleaned clothes or by finding a cleaner who uses *wet-cleaning* methods instead. Wet-cleaning is a water-based alternative to solvent-based dry cleaning that uses biodegradable detergents and a humidity-controlled drying environment to preserve "dry-clean only" clothes.

If you can't avoid dry-cleaned clothes, store them in a well-ventilated spot away from your living area (like the garage or an outdoor building), and each time they're treated, allow them to air out for several days (or weeks if time allows) before wearing them.

8. Reduce Your Exposure to Unnecessary Electromagnetic Radiation

Opt for corded and wired devices over cordless and Wi-Fi devices whenever you can. Keep all Wi-Fi transmitters away from where you work, sleep, or spend significant amounts of time. Remove unnecessary electronic gadgets from the bedroom, and do not sleep next to wireless devices unless they are completely powered down. Don't position sleeping areas next to a wall shared by large appliances like refrigerators, freezers, and electric ovens. Keep computers at arm's length and position seating areas at least six feet away from televisions. Don't keep cell phones or other wireless devices in your pockets or next to your body when they are turned on. Use a wired headset or speakerphone whenever possible. Keep calls short, and when you don't need to speak in person, send text messages instead. Use wireless devices only when the signal strength is strong. Avoid using them in transit and inside spaces enclosed by metal like elevators, subways, trains, planes, and cars, unless they can be connected to a built-in external antenna.

9. Use Plants to Clean the Air

Houseplants can act as natural air filters and greatly improve the quality of indoor air. Certain species have been shown to remove toxic compounds from indoor air:

- Snake plant (*Sansevieria trifasciata*) (Papinchak et al. 2009)

- Spider plant (*Chlorophytum comosum*) (Papinchak et al. 2009)

- English ivy (*Hedera helix*) (Yoo, Kwon, and Son 2006)

- Grape ivy (*Cissus rhombifolia*) (Yoo, Kwon, and Son 2006)

- Peace lily (*Spathiphyllum wallisii, Spathiphyllum clevelandii*) (Yoo, Kwon, and Son 2006)

- Golden pothos (*Epipremnum aureum*) (Papinchak et al. 2009)

- Weeping fig (*Ficus benjamina*) (Kim et al. 2008)

- Nephthytis (*Syngonium podophyllum*) (Yoo, Kwon, and Son 2006)

- Japanese aralia (*Fatsia japonica*) (Kim et al. 2008)

Aim for one six-inch houseplant per one hundred square feet of living area.

10. Dispose of Household Trash Responsibly

Be sure to dispose as hazardous waste any household items that contain toxic components. This includes leftover paint, solvents, automotive fluids, batteries, and all electronic items. Do not put these items into your regular trash. If they end up in landfills, the toxic chemicals they contain can pollute the environment and make their way into water and soil. Contact your local authority to learn about the disposal options in your area.

11. Use Nontoxic Furnishings and Building Supplies

If you are planning to refurnish or remodel your home, or if you're buying or building a new home, use nontoxic building materials whenever possible:

- Tiles made of stone, porcelain, glass, or ceramic

- Prefinished real hardwood furniture and flooring

- Shellac (a clear, hard finish made from resin secreted by insects)

- Low-VOC water-based (latex) paint

- Organic cotton, wool, or natural latex mattresses and mattress pads (avoid latex if you are allergic to it)

- Organic cotton fabrics, bedding, and washable rugs

- Wool carpet, which is durable and naturally fire retardant, or no carpet at all

When removing old paint or carpet, take the appropriate precautions or hire professionals to do it safely for you. After applying fresh paint indoors, allow it to *off-gas*, or release fumes, for as long as possible before spending prolonged periods of time in the area. Before installing new carpet or furniture, allow them to off-gas in an unoccupied area, like an outdoor building, for as long as possible (weeks or even months if time allows).

12. Test for Toxins

Install and maintain a carbon-monoxide detector. Have your home tested for mold, radon, and lead. Use furnace filters with a

MERV (minimum efficiency reporting value) of 7 to 9, and change them every six weeks. Clean out your air ducts and vents regularly, especially active fireplace vents. If you can't do these things yourself, hire professionals.

A Less Toxic Home

We can't completely escape environmental toxins, but we certainly can reduce our exposure. Some steps like opening the windows and leaving your shoes at the door are easy and inexpensive. Others involve more time and require more money, like researching your personal products or investing in air filters. Remember that whether you're able to follow all these recommendations or implement just one or two, every little bit helps.

chapter 7

Maintenance Plan

To permanently reverse prediabetes and stay healthy, the prediabetes detox program must be followed by a long-term maintenance plan. If you return to your previous diet and lifestyle, it's likely that prediabetes will return too. Once you've finished detoxification, resist any urges to celebrate with foods or drinks that aren't allowed on the detox diet you've been following. You aren't done with it yet. This is the time to reintroduce foods you've been avoiding and observe how they really affect your blood sugar. Going forward, your blood sugar levels will be a good predictor of your long-term success in reversing prediabetes. Testing your individual reactions to certain foods is the best way to determine what you should be eating every day. Some people can eat unprocessed whole grains or fresh fruit without raising their blood glucose levels, and others can't. We all have our own genetic and epigenetic predispositions, and only by testing your reaction to foods will you know how to tailor a healthy diet just for you.

In addition to a healthy diet, you should consider keeping some of the supplements in your regular routine. Most people benefit from taking a multivitamin/mineral formula, vitamin D, omega-3 fats in the form of fish oil (or algae oil), probiotics, and green tea in capsule form, if you don't drink it every day. After detoxification, you can reduce your dose of omega-3s to 1,000 milligrams of DHA and EPA per day. You can continue the same dosages of the multivitamin/mineral formula, vitamin D, probiotics, and green tea that you've been taking during detoxification.

You'll also want to continue many of the daily detox habits, like getting regular exercise and plenty of sleep. Later, this chapter will get more specific, and I'll offer my top ten tips for staying healthy for the rest of your life. But first, here are some guidelines for food reintroduction.

Food Reintroduction

After you finish detoxification, you will reintroduce some of the foods you've been avoiding back into your diet to determine the effects they have on your blood sugar. If any of the foods you reintroduce cause abnormally high blood sugar elevations, you'll know it's best for you to continue avoiding these foods. If the foods you reintroduce do not disrupt your blood sugar levels, you can add them back to your diet permanently.

General Guidelines

There are four important guidelines for food reintroduction:

1. Reintroduce foods in their most pure and preferably whole-food form. For example, don't reintroduce gluten by eating cookies that contain several potentially problematic ingredients. Instead, go to the source and reintroduce wheat berries.

2. Each time you reintroduce a new food, make sure it's the only change you make. If you change more than one thing at a time and you have a reaction, you won't be able to accurately determine the cause.

3. When you test a new food, eat it twice a day for three days unless you have a reaction. If the food passes the three-day test, you can add it to your diet permanently.

4. If you react to a food you've reintroduced, stop eating it immediately and wait until your morning fasting blood

sugar level has normalized and any other symptoms have cleared before you reintroduce another new food.

Remember that some of the foods you may be reintroducing should only be eaten in their organic form, including dairy products, foods that may be genetically modified (corn, soy, and Hawaiian papaya), and those that contain the most pesticide residues (apples, grapes, peaches, nectarines, and potatoes).

Step-by-Step Details

Once the detox program is over, discontinue the supplements (other than the basics) and saunas (or baths), but maintain the other lifestyle guidelines and the detox diet throughout the food reintroduction process. For the first three days post-detox, record your blood sugar levels four times each day: when you wake up in the morning (and before eating breakfast), two hours after breakfast, two hours after lunch, and two hours after dinner. After you've recorded three days of blood sugar readings, you're ready to begin reintroducing foods one at a time. Follow this food group order:

1. Unsweetened fresh and frozen fruits, besides citrus and berries

2. Dried fruits with no added oils, preservatives, or sweeteners

3. Starchy vegetables, like carrots, parsnips, pumpkin, winter squash, rutabagas, potatoes, sweet potatoes, and yams

4. Gluten-free whole grains, like corn, quinoa, brown rice, wild rice, millet, buckwheat (kasha), and amaranth

5. Whole grains that contain gluten, like wheat, barley, rye, and oatmeal (oats are naturally gluten-free but are often contaminated by cross-pollination in the field or by processing in plants that also process gluten-containing grains)

6. Two ounces of dark chocolate at a time, 72 to 85 percent dark

7. Alcohol (optional)

8. Foods you've been avoiding because you suspect sensitivities, like dairy, soy, eggs, peanuts, tree nuts, or shellfish

If a food you've been avoiding during detox isn't on this list (like sugar or flour), you should never reintroduce them. After reversing prediabetes, some people can safely resume eating certain whole foods (like fruits, root vegetables, and grains), but everyone should avoid processed foods indefinitely.

Note that it's important to reintroduce individual foods within food groups separately. That is, if apricots pass the test, you can't assume that all fruits are fine for you. You may be able to tolerate quinoa but not corn, pumpkin but not potatoes, or yogurt but not cream.

Focus on Foods You Want to Eat

If you reintroduce every single food you've been avoiding, the entire process could take months, so focus first on the foods that you want to eat regularly. (If you don't like watermelon, for example, don't bother reintroducing it.) Looking at diet from a long-term perspective, what you eat most of the time is more important than what you eat only occasionally. From time to time, you'll likely eat foods that aren't part of your ideal diet. That's okay, but when you do, be sure to limit yourself to a small portion.

There's no need to reintroduce foods that you're certain you are allergic or sensitive to. Just continue avoiding them. If you've been avoiding foods because you suspect a sensitivity or intolerance but you're not certain, follow the same guidelines to introduce them, but be on the lookout for symptoms besides blood sugar elevations. They may include headaches, congestion, skin rashes, general malaise, fatigue, and changes in mood or digestion. If you have a reaction to a food you've reintroduced, stop the food immediately and continue avoiding it.

Some people who can't tolerate dairy products made from cow's milk do very well with sheep- or goat-milk products. If you've been avoiding dairy products and you're interested in reintroducing them, consider starting with those made from sheep's milk or goat's milk before you try cow's milk. Also test different products separately (butter, cream, yogurt, cheese). You may tolerate certain forms better than others, depending on whether you have a sensitivity or intolerance, so be sure to test individually all of the foods you want to add back into your diet.

Limit Alcohol Consumption

The method for reintroducing alcohol will be slightly different. Your choices will be limited to forms of alcohol with little or no sugar: four to six ounces of dry red or white wine (flat or sparkling); or one ounce (for women) or two ounces (for men) of unsweetened pure distilled spirits, including vodka, gin, tequila, rum, brandy, cognac, or whiskey. Pure distilled spirits don't contain any carbohydrates at all unless they are mixed with soda, juice, or other mixers. Test alcohol only once per day (not twice a day) and always drink it with food, never on an empty stomach. If you wish, pour spirits over ice, add them to sodium-free seltzer water, or muddle them with citrus fruit, berries, grated ginger, or fresh mint leaves. If alcohol passes the test, you can have one drink three times each week (see the guidelines later in this chapter). Forms of alcohol you should completely avoid, now and forever, include beer, sweet and semidry wines, dessert wines, and all sweet or sweetened liquors, and mixers.

Keep a Chart

Record your blood sugar levels during the food reintroduction process and track changes related to specific foods. You can download a chart designed for this purpose at www.prediabetesdetox .com. If your blood sugar levels remain stable (similar to your control levels recorded on the first three days postdetox) when you reintroduce a new food, feel free to continue eating it. If your blood sugar readings go up two hours after consuming a new food or drink, relative to your control readings, or if your morning fasting blood sugar level goes up within forty-eight hours, stop consuming the new food or drink and wait for your blood sugar levels to return to normal before reintroducing another new food.

Long-Term Guidelines

After you've finished the prediabetes detox and determined which foods are good choices for your body, feel proud of the progress you've made. Revel in the moment and feel inspired to continue improving your health. Now that you've built a good foundation for a healthy body, it's time to start thinking about how you're going to maintain it. To help you do just that, here are my top ten recommendations for staying healthy and living a long and joyful life.

1. Avoid Toxic Foods

Maintain a diet low in sweets, starches, inflammatory fats, and toxic foods. Remember that what you eat most of the time is more important than what you eat once in a while. It's not a tragedy if you consume some of the foods or drinks listed below on rare occasion, but make them the exception rather than the rule and savor them in small amounts.

Most of the time and whenever possible, continue to avoid the following:

- Foods and beverages that contain any form of sweetener, including sugar, "natural" sweeteners, and artificial sweeteners

- Foods made from flour

- Liquid oils that have not been cold-pressed, including canola oil, soybean oil, corn oil, sunflower oil, safflower oil, cottonseed oil, peanut oil, and any toasted oil

- Cold-pressed liquid oils and raw nuts and seeds stored at room temperature

- Trans fats, hydrogenated or partially hydrogenated fats and oils, and interesterified fats and oils

- Deep-fried foods, including chips and French fries

- Roasted nuts (unless you toast them yourself in a dry skillet over low heat until just fragrant and then eat them right away)

- Meat, eggs, and dairy products from grain-fed animals

- Processed meats, including hot dogs, pepperoni, salami, bologna, Spam, sliced deli meat, and sausage (unless it's homemade)

- Low-fat and fat-free dairy products

- Butter substitutes like margarine and vegetable oil spreads

- Egg substitutes

- Fish with high levels of environmental contaminants, including tuna, tilapia, Chilean sea bass, flounder, snapper, sturgeon, and swordfish (for links to the most up-to-date information, visit www.prediabetesdetox .com)

- The Dirty Dozen Plus foods unless they are organic (see list in chapter 3)

- Nonorganic foods that may be genetically modified: corn, soy, canola oil, dairy products, sugar, cottonseed oil, Hawaiian papaya, zucchini, or yellow squash

- Fruits processed into jams, jellies, syrups, and concentrates

- Processed soy products

- Foods and beverages in contact with plastic (including epoxy-lined food containers like cans), polystyrene (Styrofoam), and nonstick surfaces

- Milk, juice, and soft drinks, whether naturally or artificially sweetened

Buy the best quality food you can afford. Foods at the top of the food chain usually contain the most toxins, so if you have to prioritize, it's more important to eat clean animal products than organic produce.

2. Eat Balanced Meals and Skip Snacks

Eat protein, healthy fat, and green vegetables with every meal, and avoid snacking between meals. Choose foods on the prediabetes detox diet and those you introduced that didn't cause problems. If you'll be eating fruits, starchy vegetables, or whole grains, remember to limit yourself to a half-cup serving of these foods per meal or per day. In general, half of each meal should be green or fibrous vegetables, one quarter should be protein, one quarter should be other foods on your list and your meal should include at least one source of healthy fat. Continue to season foods with cinnamon, ginger, cayenne, garlic, onions, fenugreek, cumin, turmeric, black pepper, parsley, and cilantro. Continue to eat fermented foods regularly. Continue to drink mostly water and unsweetened tea. If you drink coffee, have it unsweetened and limit yourself to eight ounces of brewed coffee or one ounce of espresso per day, regular or decaffeinated by the Swiss-water method.

3. Limit Your Alcohol Intake

Don't drink every day; or, if you find that alcohol disrupts your blood sugar, don't drink at all. If your blood sugar balance permits it, you can have up to three drinks each week when you follow these rules:

1. Never drink alcohol on an empty stomach. Only drink alcohol with meals.

2. Do not drink alcohol after 9:00 p.m. or within two hours of bedtime.

3. Have only one drink of four to six ounces of wine or one (for women) or two (for men) ounces of unsweetened pure

distilled spirits (vodka, gin, tequila, rum, brandy, cognac, or whiskey).

4. Never mix alcohol with soda, juice, or other sweet mixers.

4. Exercise and Sweat

Break a sweat with a sauna or bath and at least three hours of exercise each week. Once your blood sugar is under control and your fasting levels are consistently below eighty for three months, you can reduce your exercise from five hours per week to three. Continue to incorporate all three forms of exercise (aerobic, strengthening, and stretching) and to spend at least one hour each week (divided into more than one session) on strengthening exercises. Practice interval training at least twice each week and always warm up before exercise and cool down afterward. Remember, you'll need to exercise forever.

5. Get Good Sleep

Get plenty of sleep, at least eight hours each night in the summer and nine hours each night in the winter. Adequate sleep helps regulate blood sugar and fat metabolism, normalizes stress hormones, and increases the natural production of serotonin. See chapter 5 for tips on improving your sleep.

6. Get Natural Sunlight

Get ten to twenty minutes of natural sunlight every day, preferably first thing in the morning. Get up as close to sunrise as possible and go outside as soon as you can. Exposing your skin to natural morning sunlight improves sleep patterns, helps regulate blood sugar and fat metabolism, normalizes stress hormones, and increases the natural production of serotonin. Avoid midday sun and intense or excessive sun exposure. Don't leave your skin exposed long enough that you develop a sunburn. If you use sunscreen, understand that it prevents sunburn but not skin damage.

Take advantage of your time outside to maintain physical contact with the earth's conductive surfaces. Go barefoot if you can on grass, sand, dirt, gravel, or concrete surfaces, or while wading in natural water sources. If you can't be barefoot, wearing leather-soled shoes is the next best thing.

7. Keep a Regular Schedule

Wake up, eat meals, and go to bed at the same times each day. Our bodies are sensitive to our daily routines. Eating on an irregular schedule and sleeping a different number of hours or the same number of hours at different times can disrupt your circadian rhythm and the hormones that control appetite, blood sugar, and fat metabolism. The more regular your schedule, the better your body will work. As much as you can, keep regular hours for sleeping, waking, eating, and exercising.

8. Relax and Be Happy

Relax every day and have good sex every week. Mental and emotional health plays a big role in physical health. Regular relaxation and pleasurable sexual activity, either alone or with a partner, can boost serotonin levels and normalize stress hormones, helping our bodies better regulate blood sugar. So take time to relax and do things that bring you joy. Studies show that happy people have lower levels of stress hormones and lower blood pressure (Steptoe and Wardle 2005). Also, connect with others and make time to nurture relationships. If you don't have at least five good friends, meet more. A 2010 analysis of nearly 150 studies found that friendships have just as much impact on our risk of dying as body mass index, physical activity, alcohol consumption, and even cigarette smoking (Holt-Lunstad, Smith, and Layton 2010).

9. Detox Twice a Year

Doing a detox is a great way to give your body a tune-up. Because we're regularly exposed to environmental toxins, it only makes sense

to regularly remove them. If you're using detox as health maintenance, it's best done during the spring and fall, times of natural transition. I usually avoid detox in the winter, as colder temperatures and
shorter days make our bodies more likely to store fat, while warmer
weather and longer days make it easier to burn fat and detoxify.

10. Partner With a Doctor

At the end of the prediabetes detox program, your fasting blood
sugar levels should be consistently below eighty milligrams per
deciliter.

If they aren't there yet and you've done the detox for eight weeks,
you should make an appointment with a naturopathic doctor. You
may require an even stricter diet, so consider eliminating all fruit
(including berries and citrus), dark chocolate, stevia (even in small
amounts), and dairy products (if you haven't already). You may be
taking a medication that predisposes you to prediabetes (like cholesterol-lowering statins, blood pressure–lowering beta blockers and
diuretics, or anti-inflammatory drugs like glucocorticoids) when
effective alternatives exist. Or you may have underlying conditions
that need to be addressed.

Naturopathic physicians have a holistic and integrative approach.
They are trained in both Western medicine and natural therapies
like diet, exercise, detoxification, and natural medicines. Several
options exist for reversing prediabetes when detoxification and
changes in diet and lifestyle aren't enough, but what is right for one
person isn't right for everyone. It's important to find the best fit for
you. Naturopathic doctors look at the whole person, tailor treatments to meet individual needs, and use the least invasive therapies
to correct underlying imbalances that may be preventing you from
getting well. To learn more about naturopathic medicine and find
an ND in your area, visit www.prediabetesdetox.com.

Once your fasting blood sugar levels have been consistently
below eighty for three months, you should see your doctor to repeat
lab tests for fasting glucose, insulin, hemoglobin A1C, vitamin D,
and any other tests that were abnormal before you started the prediabetes detox. My generalized recommendations end there. Studies

show that screening tests and health checkups don't reduce rates of disease or death (Krogsbøll et al. 2012) and may even make unnecessary treatments more likely, so I don't recommend asking your doctor for an entire battery of tests that you may not even need. It's more important to partner with a doctor you trust, who can make recommendations for testing and treatment based on your state of health and your risk factors for illness.

Summary

There is great wisdom in the old adage that if you do what you've always done, you'll get what you've always got. So seize this opportunity to make a fresh start, and practice these guidelines to maintain good health going forward.

chapter 8

Prediabetes Detox Recipes

Amidst our busy lives, we do everything possible to spend less time on daily chores like cooking. But what we really should be doing is spending more time in the kitchen. Cooking nourishing meals is one the easiest and most effective ways to keep ourselves and our families in good health. According to a study from the National Institutes of Health, people who cook at home live longer than people who don't, regardless of their knowledge of nutrition and physical ability to shop for food and prepare meals. Researchers found that people who cooked at home at least five times per week were 47 percent more likely to be alive ten years later, but even people who cooked less frequently saw benefits. The more frequently they cooked, the longer they lived (Chen et al. 2012).

Think of cooking dinner as a time to relax and wind down from your day. Make it especially productive by planning or preparing a healthy lunch for tomorrow. If you live alone, turn on some music and use this time to nurture yourself. Invite your friends and neighbors to cook with you or share the delicious meals you make. If you live with your family, take the opportunity to connect with them and get everyone involved, especially your kids, if you have any. Children are always more likely to eat foods they prepare themselves, so teach them early on to make simple and healthy dishes like salads. They can wash lettuce leaves, tear them up with clean hands or cut them up with scissors, make their own vinaigrette by shaking up a few ingredients in a glass jar with a tight-fitting lid, and toss everything together. Cooking healthy meals is an important life skill, and the sooner you start, the healthier you'll be.

In my practice, I see a big difference in the overall health of people who cook meals from scratch and those who live on fast food, prepared meals, and restaurant fare—which is extremely common in Manhattan, where apartments are tiny, kitchens can be poorly equipped, ovens are used for storage instead of cooking, and there are more restaurants per capita than any other city in the United States. But the number one thing that most people can do to improve their health is to prepare their own food. Some of my patients are reluctant to try, but they soon learn that cooking from scratch is easier and more fun than they imagined, that buying groceries is cheaper than paying for prepared foods, that meals they cook themselves taste much better than foods found elsewhere, and that the health benefits speak for themselves. Certainly there can be a place in our lives for occasional prepared foods and restaurant meals. After all, what we do most of the time is much more important than what we do once in a while. But during detox, diet is critically important, so if you aren't accustomed to cooking, it's time to spend more time in the kitchen.

Preparing healthy meals is really a three-step process. You have to plan the meals you want to make, gather your ingredients, and then do the actual cooking. This chapter will support your success in all three areas. First it will make suggestions for meal planning and seeking out healthy ingredients. Then it will introduce the top twelve detox foods and give you recipes and serving suggestions to get you started. You'll be able to find more recipes at www.prediabe tesdetox.com.

Meal Planning

To plan detox-friendly meals, consider creative alternatives to common cuisine. Have soup or salad instead of sandwiches. Take whatever you would put inside your sandwich and put it on top of a big green salad. Instead of preparing rice, couscous, or pasta, finely chop cauliflower (florets and tender leaves and stems) in a food processor, sauté it with a little coconut oil or olive oil, and season it with sea salt. (I call it "cauliflower couscous.") Instead of making mashed potatoes, cook and purée cauliflower, white beans, chickpeas, or artichoke hearts. You can season them the same way you would potatoes, with butter, salt, pepper, and heavy cream or bone broth. Instead of eating toast or cereal or pancakes for breakfast, think outside the box. If chicken soup or wild salmon and broccoli make a healthy dinner or lunch, they also make a healthy breakfast. You don't have to eat traditional breakfast foods for breakfast, and you don't have to eat traditional dinner foods only for dinner. Try having dinner for breakfast instead.

Another strategy for planning healthy meals is to learn how to make some basic condiments with whole foods instead of processed ingredients, without any of the additives common in store-bought varieties. Such condiments as salsa, pesto, tapenade, compound butter (butter mixed with ingredients like garlic, herbs, citrus zest, or blue cheese), Dijon-style mustard, aioli, and real mayonnaise (which is just egg yolks and olive oil, seasoned with a little lemon juice and salt) can go with several dishes.

If it's hard for you to find the time to cook every day, spend one of your days off preparing some food to eat during the upcoming week or to store in your freezer. Homemade condiments that have a good amount of fat, like compound butter, pesto, and tapenade, freeze well. After you roast a chicken, use leftover meat for salads, soups, and stir-fries. Or freeze the leftover meat for future use. (Leftover chicken is so versatile that you may want to roast an extra bird while you're at it.) When you make a pot of soup, double the recipe and store some in the freezer. If you mix up veggie burgers or Moroccan Lamb Sliders (the recipe is in this chapter), wrap them individually and freeze them for another day (thaw them in the fridge the night before you want to eat them).

If you need ideas for turning individual recipes into well-balanced meals, visit www.prediabetesdetox.com. I've put together three different week-long menus, one for omnivores, one for vegetarians, and a third for people following a dairy-free diet.

Grocery Shopping

Making healthy meals from scratch is easiest in a well-stocked kitchen. Visit www.prediabetesdetox.com for detailed lists of kitchen staples you'll want to keep in your pantry, fridge, and freezer.

Produce

Fresh produce is best when it's locally grown and harvested in season. If you can, plant a garden and grow your own vegetables, fruits, and herbs. (It's a great way to connect with the earth and get regular exercise as well as your daily dose of sunshine.) If you can't plant a garden outdoors, consider planting a window garden. You can grow fresh herbs and leafy greens in almost any sunny windowsill. Visit www.prediabetesdetox.com for more information about container gardening.

The next best thing to growing your own is getting it from a local farmer. Shop at the farmers' market or join a community-supported agriculture (CSA) group. CSA shares offer farm-fresh foods every week during harvest season and usually include a variety of vegetables. Some shares also offer fruits, flowers, herbs, dairy products, and pasture-raised eggs. Produce is always freshly picked and usually organic (check with the farmer). Visit www.prediabetes detox.com to find farmers' markets and CSAs near you.

If you are able, preserve fresh produce in season, when fully ripe and bursting with nutrients, and eat it all year long. Freeze berries, can tomatoes, preserve lemons, ferment cabbage into sauerkraut or vegetables into kimchi, and pickle cucumbers, beets, green beans, and onions. If you shy away from preserving your own food because canning seems complicated or freezer space is limited, know that there are lots of other preservation techniques. An excellent resource is *Preserving Food without Freezing or Canning: Traditional Techniques Using Salt, Oil, Sugar, Alcohol, Vinegar, Drying, Cold Storage, and Lactic Fermentation* by the gardeners and farmers of Terre Vivante, a nonprofit association based in France.

If you buy preserved foods, look for those in glass jars or BPA-free and phthalate-free cans. Companies like Muir Glen and Trader Joe's use BPA-free cans, and it's not difficult to find foods stored in glass jars, like tomato purée (sometimes called *passata*), olives, pickles, capers, sauerkraut, kimchi, preserved lemons, and dried herbs and spices.

Fish and Seafood

If you have access to a fish and seafood market, learn how to identify freshness (no smell, clear eyes, firm flesh) and make friends with your local fishmonger. Lots of small and inexpensive fish and seafood species are available year-round. Learn how to cook and eat whole fish (for instructions on how to remove most of the bones easily and in one piece, visit www.prediabetesdetox.com) and use the bones to make your own fish stock. If you live by freshwater, check with your local authorities before eating what's caught there, since most fish from US lakes and rivers should be avoided due to a build-up of environmental toxins.

If you don't have access to fresh seafood, frozen or canned wild Alaskan salmon is a great alternative. It's available year-round and costs much less than fresh salmon, which is not only expensive but in season just a few months each year. Canned herring, trout, sardines, and anchovies are also inexpensive and available year-round. Look for fish in BPA-free cans, which are available at Trader Joe's and online from Vital Choice seafood (find these links at www.prediabetesdetox.com).

Meat and Animal Products

Because animals are at the top of the food chain, they usually contain more toxins than plant foods, so always buy the best quality meats and animal products you can afford. Pasture-raised and grass-fed meat is usually more expensive than grain-fed meat, but there are ways to incorporate it into your diet without breaking the bank.

Find a Local Farmer

Buying from the source makes the most economic sense. When you meet the people who grow your food, they're usually happy to tell you how they did it. Find these farmers at your local farmers' market.

Buy in Bulk

Some farmers offer animal shares, or the option to buy a certain portion of an animal, or you may find other people in your community who will share the cost of a whole or partial cow, lamb, or pig. You'll get a lot of meat at once, but if you store it properly (airtight in your freezer), it will last a long time.

Buy the Whole Animal

When it comes to smaller animals like chickens, ducks, and rabbits, buy the whole thing rather than pieces. Learn how to cut up the meat, or ask your butcher to do it for you.

Buy the Cheaper Cuts

Ground meat, tougher cuts like shoulders and shanks, and parts like the tongue, heart, and liver are less expensive than prime cuts, and when properly cooked, they can make some of the most succulent and delicious dishes. Organ meats are full of nutrients, and they're often overlooked.

You can find a recipe for homemade paté at www.prediabetes detox.com. For more information and ideas on cooking organ meats, less commonly consumed parts like tongue and tripe, and meats like rabbit and pheasant, read *The Whole Beast: Nose to Tail Eating* by Fergus Henderson. Cook roasts (preferably bone-in), shanks, and joints in a warm oven (between 250 and 300°F) for several hours. Use ground meat to make chili, meatballs (serve large ones with tomato sauce and add small ones to soups), meatloaf (use an egg as a binder instead of bread crumbs), patties and sliders (serve them with a salad instead of buns), and stuffed vegetables (like tomatoes, peppers, and eggplant). Make your own preservative-free sausage by combining ground meat with seasonings like sea salt, freshly ground pepper, garlic, parsley, fennel seeds, allspice, nutmeg, paprika, cayenne, caraway, cumin, thyme, oregano, and/or red wine vinegar (find a recipe at www.prediabetesdetox.com).

Get Wild Game

If you hunt or know someone who does, jump at the opportunity to add wild game to your diet. For ideas on cooking wild game (as well as foraged foods), read *Hunt, Gather, Cook: Finding the Forgotten Feast* by Hank Shaw, and *Girl Hunter: Revolutionizing the Way We Eat, One Hunt at a Time* by Georgia Pellegrini.

Use Meat as a Condiment

Meat doesn't have to be the star of the show. It's better to eat smaller quantities of good-quality meat than larger quantities of poor-quality meat. (Actually, it's best not to eat poor-quality meat at all.) Learn to use meat like a condiment, as a way to add flavor and texture to vegetable-based meals like stir-fries, soups, salads, and stuffed vegetables.

Eat More Eggs

Technically, eggs aren't meat, but they are a less expensive pasture-raised animal product and a great source of nutrients, protein, and omega-3 fatty acids. To get all of the benefits, you have to eat all of the egg, not just the white. Eggs are incredibly versatile, and they can be eaten for any meal. They can be poached, fried, or scrambled (alone or with onions, garlic, leafy greens, fresh herbs, or cheese). They can be eaten as omelets, frittatas, and crustless quiches.

They can be soft- or hard-boiled, then peeled, rinsed, and added to salads or served as a starter (cut them in half and top them with anchovies or capers, freshly chopped dill or parsley, and a drizzle of olive oil). Boiled eggs make a great snack because they're portable, they don't need to be refrigerated, and they can be eaten at room temperature with just a little sprinkle of sea salt. Eggs can also be baked with vegetables like sautéed spinach or leftover ratatouille (make indentations in the cooked vegetables, crack an egg into each one, and bake until the whites are firmly set).

Thanks to consumer demand, it's becoming easier in many areas to find healthy foods, including organic produce, organic and grass-fed dairy products, pasture-raised and grass-fed meats and eggs, and wild Alaskan salmon. We certainly have a long way to go, but steady progress is being made.

Top Twelve Detox Foods

There are lots of good foods included in the prediabetes detox diet, but some certainly stand out. The most important foods for detox are artichokes; beets; berries; broccoli and cauliflower; brussels sprouts and cabbages; green leafy vegetables; mushrooms; nuts, coconut, and cacao; fermented foods; wild Alaskan salmon; pasture-raised poultry; and grass-fed meat. Chapter 3 covered the many benefits of eating these healthy foods. This chapter includes serving suggestions and at least one recipe for each food. You can find more recipes at www.prediabetesdetox.com.

1. Artichokes

Get fresh artichokes when they're in season or find them frozen year-round. If they are fresh, trim them down to the choke to use in recipes, or steam them whole until the petals can be pulled out easily. Dip each one in vinaigrette and eat the tender edible parts. When you get to the heart, remove the choke, quarter the heart and stem, and eat them with vinaigrette too. You can add fresh or frozen artichoke hearts to soups or stirfries. Add cooked artichoke hearts to salads, or marinate them with red wine vinegar, olive oil, fresh or dried herbs, minced garlic, lemon zest, sea salt, and freshly ground pepper. See recipe: Artichoke Olive Tapinade.

2. Beets

Look for beets that still have their green leafy tops, and eat the green parts too. Cook them like you would kale or any other green leafy vegetable. Beets come in several varieties, so feel free to experiment if you're used to the red ones.

I like to toss grated yellow beets into salads or serve them as a starter, drizzled with vinaigrette and garnished with cilantro leaves. Chioggia beets, with their distinctive pattern of concentric red and white rings, are best appreciated sliced thin (using a mandoline) and eaten raw in salads, as their colors fade when you cook them.

You can also use beets to make soups like borscht. Use them in place of carrots and other root vegetables in other kinds of soup (if you don't want soups to turn purple, use golden beets) and alongside roasted meats. See recipe: Roasted Beet Salad

3. Berries

Berries can be eaten raw by themselves, added to salads, mixed into yogurt, or blended into smoothies. But they also make delicious and nutritious savory sauces. (Simply thaw frozen raspberries, retaining the juices, and gently stir in salt, pepper, and a dash of balsamic vinegar.) Their tart fruit flavor pairs especially well with fattier meats like duck and stronger flavors like salmon, pheasant, lamb, and venison. They also can rescue leaner meats that sometimes turn out dry, like turkey and pork, and they can dress up meats that could use more flavor, like chicken. See recipe: Morning Detox Smoothie.

4. Broccoli and Cauliflower

Broccoli, broccoli rabe, and cauliflower are actually flowers. Some of their healthy compounds are destroyed by boiling, so eat these vegetables steamed until crisp-tender, or consume them raw (unless you have thyroid problems). You can eat the stems of broccoli and cauliflower as well as the flowers. Broccoli stems are tender and sweet after you trim away the bottom and tough outer layers (use a vegetable peeler or sharp knife). Raw broccoli and cauliflower florets and tender stems go well in salads, or you can dip them in hummus. Add them to curries and stir-fries. Make cream of broccoli soup. If you need a quick side dish, steam chunks of broccoli or cauliflower, season with salt, and toss with butter or drizzle with olive oil or vinaigrette. See recipe: Cauliflower With Walnut Pesto.

5. Brussels Sprouts and Cabbages

Cabbage is the biggest bargain in produce. It's inexpensive and it's the only green leafy vegetable on the Clean Fifteen list. There are lots of varieties of cabbage: green, red, Savoy, Napa, bok choy, tatsoi, and brussels sprouts. Toss brussels sprouts with melted ghee and roast them in a hot oven (400°F) until golden brown. Add cabbage to soups, stir-fries, or curry. Braise wedges of cabbage with a bit of bone broth at a low temperature (325°F) for a couple of hours until tender and sweet. Blanch large cabbage leaves in boiling water, and then stuff with a mixture of ground meat, vegetables, herbs, and grated Parmesan cheese. Roll the leaves up like burritos, and bake in tomato sauce (puréed tomatoes, onions, and herbs) until warm throughout. Stir grated garlic into the sauce just before serving. See recipe: Brussels Sprouts Sauté.

6. Green Leafy Vegetables

Green leafy vegetables are good sources of fiber, vitamins, minerals, antioxidants, and chlorophyll. Salad greens are tender and easily eaten raw, while winter greens, including kale, Swiss chard, beet greens, collard greens, mustard greens, and mature spinach, are tougher and more bitter. They can be rolled up and thinly cut into ribbons for salads, but they're usually eaten cooked.

Winter greens can be used like any other vegetable in stir-fries, curries, and soups. You can make creamed greens by cooking them until tender and puréeing them with sea salt, freshly ground pepper, and a dash of heavy cream. Or make kale chips by removing the ribs, tearing the leaves in pieces, tossing them with olive oil and sea salt, and oven-roasting them in at a low temperature until crisp.

Salad greens come in all shades, shapes, and sizes: arugula, butter (Boston) lettuce, endive, frisée, escarole, red and green leaf lettuces, mâche, mizuna, romaine, watercress, and radicchio. Young versions of winter greens are also good in salads; try baby spinach, baby chard, and baby kale.

Salads can be minimal or complex, depending on the ingredients available and the amount of time and energy you have. At the very least, my salads usually contain some sort of greens and thinly sliced red onions, shallots, or scallions. They often contain chopped raw nuts and vegetables like bell peppers, celery, fennel, cucumbers, or radishes, thinly sliced on a mandoline. (You can chop vegetables by hand, but a mandoline can slice them thinner, which makes tough vegetables easier to eat, and it can slice them more uniformly. You also may find using a mandolin quicker than using a knife, depending your knife skills.) If the salad itself is the main course, be sure to add a good source of protein like shredded chicken or turkey, thinly sliced steak, sautéed tempeh strips, cooked chickpeas, or hard- or soft-boiled eggs. You can also add roasted red peppers, olives, marinated artichoke hearts, or crumbled feta cheese, goat cheese, or blue cheese. See recipes: Everyday Salad with Homemade Vinaigrette; Kale with Anchovies, Lemon, and Garlic.

Salad Prep

Salads sound easy to make, but there are some essential steps to follow if you want a crispy and perfectly seasoned salad.

Clean the greens when you bring them home. Discard any damaged leaves and submerge the rest in a generous amount of cold water inside a large basin or salad spinner. Swish the leaves around to loosen any debris, and soak for two or three minutes, or longer if they're wilted.

Rinse each leaf individually, taking care to remove any dirt. (Nothing spoils a salad like biting into something sandy.)

Use a salad spinner to remove excess water from the leaves, so they are neither too dry nor too wet. If you allow them to become completely dry, they may wilt. If you leave them too wet, they will spoil faster, and the extra moisture will water down your salad dressing. As an alternative to a salad spinner, use two large clean towels. Place the lettuce leaves inside one towel, gather the corners and edges, and spin it around until most of the water from the leaves has been absorbed. Arrange the leaves in a single layer on top of the second (dry) towel, roll it up, and store in the fridge.

After you've cleaned and dried your salad leaves, allow them to chill inside the fridge for several hours. Toss them with salad dressing only just before you eat them (or they may become soggy).

7. Mushrooms

Edible mushrooms support detoxification by reducing inflammation, enhancing antioxidant activity, and protecting insulin-producing cells in the pancreas. They're also good for blood sugar control, for they inhibit the absorption of glucose and improve insulin sensitivity (Lo and Wasser 2011). Mushrooms are one of the Clean Fifteen least contaminated produce items, and widely available at farmers' markets and in grocery stores. Look for shiitake, maitake, portobello, crimini, oyster, and button mushrooms. When you can't find them fresh, buy them dried. Dried porcini mushrooms can be expensive, but dried shiitakes are much more affordable and readily available in Asian markets. Dried mushrooms can be reconstituted in hot water for soups, stews, roasts, and sauces, or they can be ground into a powder (with an electric grinder) and added as a seasoning to almost anything. Dried mushroom powder is especially good in spice rubs for meats like beef and lamb.

Thinly sliced mushroom caps can be sautéed with butter, ghee, or olive oil and seasoned with sea salt for a simple side dish. (Reserve the stems for bone broth.) Large mushrooms caps can be stuffed (with ground meat or homemade sausage cooked with onions and pulsed in a food processor with garlic, herbs, and walnuts), then baked until cooked through. Make mushroom gravy by sautéing mushrooms with butter or rendered chicken or duck fat, sliced onions, garlic, and herbs, then puréeing with bone broth until smooth. Broil portobello mushroom caps by placing them gill side up on a baking sheet, drizzling them with olive oil, sprinkling them with sea salt, and cooking them under a broiler until the gills become browned and crispy. Slice and serve them for a simple side dish, or add them to salads, scrambled eggs, or miso soup. Or, fill them with sautéed spinach, top them with cheese, bake until they are cooked through, and serve them with tomato sauce. See recipe: Medicinal Mushroom Soup.

8. Nuts, Coconut, and Cacao

I recommend soaking nuts before you eat them. Soaking increases the activity of beneficial enzymes, neutralizes phytic acid (which inhibits the absorption of minerals), makes proteins easier to digest and nutrients easier to absorb, and converts starches and fats to proteins and vitamins. Soak nuts by covering them generously with filtered water and setting them aside at room temperature for 24 hours. Add more water as needed to keep them covered as they expand. After soaking, you can use them wet, allow them to dry at room temperature, dry them in a dehydrator, or oven-dry them at a very low temperature (no more than 150°F) for 12 to 24 hours. Store all nuts in the fridge or freezer.

Toss whole or chopped nuts into salads. Purée them into soups or sauces as a natural thickener. Make a Spanish Romesco sauce by roasting red peppers and tomatoes and puréeing them with soaked almonds, garlic, olive oil, salt, pepper, and cayenne or paprika. Add cashews to stir-fries, smoothies, soups, and curries.

Coconut is a variety of nut, and coconut milk is made from coconuts. Canned coconut milk can be found in most grocery stores, and frozen varieties are often available in Asian markets. Check the ingredients label and avoid products with additives like sweeteners, stabilizers (xanthan gum, carrageenan, guar gum), and chemical preservatives. The brand Aroy-D from Thailand makes coconut milk with only two ingredients: coconut extract and water. You can also make your own coconut milk if you have fresh coconut (blend chunks of the white flesh with water and strain out the solids).

Like nuts, cacao beans are the reproductive parts of the cacao plant. Roasted and fermented, they're called *nibs*. Cocoa nibs are crushed to make chocolate liquor, which is separated into cocoa butter and cocoa mass, which is crushed into cocoa powder. These components, in varying amounts, are used to make chocolate. Chocolate also contains sugar in varying amounts. The darker the chocolate, the more cocoa powder it contains, the less sugar it contains, and the more health benefits it has. Studies show that small amounts of dark chocolate rich in cocoa powder reduce insulin resistance and increase insulin sensitivity (Grassi et al. 2005). Eaten in small amounts, the benefits of dark chocolate thus outweigh the risks of the small amount of sugar it contains, but only *in small amounts*. In large amounts, the risks will outweigh the benefits, and dark chocolate becomes a bad idea for both detox and prediabetes. Remember that during the prediabetes detox program, you're allowed only one ounce per day of 85 percent dark chocolate. It can be hard to find good chocolate that is 85 percent dark, as many varieties are dry, flavorless, or bitter. Try Green & Blacks, Valrhona, or the Dark Lover's Chocolate Bar from Trader Joe's. See recipe: Dark Chocolate Clusters

Selecting the Healthiest Chocolate

Not all chocolate is good for you, and the ingredients make all the difference. The best bars have a high cocoa content, which makes them a good source of the polyphenols, flavonols, proanthocyanidins, and catechins shown to reduce the risk of diabetes (along with cardiovascular disease and cancer). Follow these guidelines to select the healthiest chocolate:

1. Avoid white chocolate. It doesn't contain any cocoa powder at all.

2. Avoid milk chocolate. It contains less cocoa powder and more sugar than dark varieties.

3. Look for products that list cocoa powder, cocoa butter, cocoa mass, and/or chocolate liquor before sugar. Even dark chocolate contains some sugar, but it should be one of the last ingredients.

4. Make sure that the only fat listed in the ingredients is cocoa butter.

5. Avoid chocolate that contains Dutch-process, or alkalinized, cocoa powder. It is made from cacao beans that have been treated with an alkalizing agent to neutralize natural acidity. Alkalizing agents destroy healthy antioxidants, so always opt for chocolate made with natural unsweetened cocoa powder instead.

6. Avoid products that contain agave, artificial sweeteners, corn syrup, vegetable oil, and hydrogenated or partially hydrogenated ingredients of any kind.

9. Fermented Foods

The fermented foods you can eat during the prediabetes detox include vinegar, lacto-fermented pickles, capers, olives, sauerkraut, kimchi, umeboshi, tempeh, miso, tamari, fish sauce, and cacao nibs. If you're not avoiding dairy products, you can also have yogurt, aged and ripened cheeses, and cultured butter.

To incorporate these foods into your diet, you can garnish meals with pickled vegetables and serve sauerkraut as a side dish (it goes especially well with fattier meats like slow-roasted pork, duck legs, and homemade sausage). You can even learn to make your own sauerkraut, yogurt, and pickled vegetables if you're interested (*Nourishing Traditions*, by Sally Fallon, is a great resource for simple and straightforward recipes). If you're not dairy-free, add some yogurt to your morning smoothie or have it with berries for dessert. Add some cheese to your salad or scrambled eggs, or serve a cheese course for dessert. Make miso soup by stirring miso paste into hot water or bone broth and adding seaweed, thinly sliced mushrooms, and thinly sliced scallions. To make miso soup a main course, poach some sablefish or salmon in the broth before you add the other ingredients. You can use tamari and fish sauce to season curries or sautéed vegetables. Tempeh can be crumbled into vegetarian chili or cut into cubes and added to stir-fries. I like to slice tempeh into thin strips and sauté in coconut oil or ghee until the strips are browned on both sides. I drizzle them with tamari while they're hot and eat them, as is, or add them to salads. Tempeh can also be used to make home-made veggie burgers. See recipe: Thai Curry With Tempeh and Mixed Vegetables.

10. Wild Alaskan Salmon

Fresh wild Alaskan salmon is a luxury to enjoy whenever you can. The rest of the time, look for wild Alaskan salmon frozen or canned. Frozen salmon usually comes vacuum-packed in plastic, so be sure to remove the wrapping before you thaw it, ideally overnight in the fridge.

Wild salmon has less fat than farm-raised salmon, and it can dry out if you cook it too quickly or for too long, so the most important thing to remember when you're cooking wild salmon is to not over-cook it. Fresh and thawed frozen salmon can be sautéed, poached, roasted, or cured. Curing your own salmon with sea salt is easy, and it's a healthy alternative to smoked salmon (go to www.prediabetes detox.com for a simple recipe). I usually prefer to slow-roast it at a low temperature while I toss a salad and make a sauce.

Leftover cooked, flaked salmon and canned salmon can be added to salads, made into chowder, stirred into miso soup, or scrambled into eggs. You can also make salmon cakes (similar to crab cakes) by mixing cooked salmon (with the skin and bones finely chopped and mixed in too) with finely chopped aromatic vegetables like onions, celery, red bell peppers, and mushrooms; fresh herbs like dill, parsley, and cilantro; seasonings like grated ginger, garlic, and lemon zest; and bread-free binders like ground walnuts and a beaten egg. Form the mixture into patties and sauté in coconut oil or ghee. See recipe: Blackened Salmon.

11. Pasture-Raised Poultry

Eat skin-on, bone-in cuts of meat whenever you can, and avoid leaner ones like boneless skinless chicken breasts. Buy your poultry in one piece, if possible. I recommend investing in sharp kitchen shears and a boning knife, and learning how to cut it up yourself when you don't want to roast the entire bird. Or you can ask your butcher to do it for you. Always season poultry with salt inside and out before you cook it to allow the seasoning to penetrate throughout, about ½ teaspoon of salt per pound of meat, at least 8 hours in advance and ideally 24 to 48 hours before cooking.

Low-Sodium Diets Are Ineffective

People with high blood pressure are advised to eat a low-sodium diet, but studies show that it doesn't really make a difference. In a review of 167 studies investigating the effects of low-sodium diets on blood pressure, researchers found that they made almost no difference, lowering blood pressure by only 1 percent in people with normal blood pressure and by only 3.5 percent in people with high blood pressure (Graudal, Hubeck-Graudal, and Jurgens 2011).

Most of the sodium in our diet comes from processed foods, and it's still important to avoid those, but don't be afraid to season whole foods with salt. Just don't go overboard.

As with all meats, bring poultry to room temperature before you start cooking. Once it's finished, save any rendered fat for high-temperature cooking and use it in place of ghee in almost any recipe (skim the fat off the top with a spoon, or use a fat separator, let it cool, and store it in an airtight container in the fridge). You can use the pan juices to make a quick sauce. Pan sauces are easy, fast, and delicious, and they leave a mostly clean pan, which makes washing up easy too. Just deglaze the pan with bone broth, cognac, brandy, or wine that's good enough to drink, reduce it by half, and stir in some fresh herbs, a spoonful of mustard, or a splash of heavy cream. Save the bones, gizzard, and heart (but not the liver) to make bone broth. The heart and gizzard can also be sautéed and added to a green salad. Use the liver to make paté (go to www.prediabetesdetox.com for a recipe) or serve it as a starter, lightly sautéed with butter, ghee, or rendered fat and drizzled with balsamic vinegar.

The best eggs come from chickens raised on pasture. If you can't find pasture-raised eggs, the next best choice is organic eggs high in omega-3s. These do come from grain-fed chickens, but at least they're pesticide-free and higher in healthy fat. Always cook eggs low and slow to prevent the cholesterol in the yolk from oxidizing and whites from getting tough. See recipes: Bone Broth; Braised Chicken Legs with Olives and Lemon.

12. Grass-Fed Meat

Meat should always be cooked low and slow too. When over-cooked, cooked at temperatures above 300°F, or cooked over an open flame, toxic compounds called polycyclic aromatic hydrocarbons (PAHs) and heterocyclic amines (HCAs) are created. (This applies to all animal proteins, including fish and seafood, but not to plant-based proteins.) Fortunately, studies show that certain foods, including rosemary, olive oil, onions, and garlic, can decrease the formation of PAHs and HCAs when these foods are used for marinating and cooking (Persson et al. 2003). Follow these guidelines to reduce your intake of toxic compounds in meats:

1. Cook tender cuts of meat like steaks quickly over high heat until rare or medium rare. Cook tougher cuts like roasts at or below 300°F for several hours.

2. Don't eat well-done meats unless they've been cooked low and slow.

3. Avoid smoked and charred meats.

4. Avoid meats cooked directly over a flame or hot coals. When grilling, choose leaner cuts of meat that cook quickly and drip less fat. You can cook them near hot coals but not directly over them.

5. Marinate or cook meats with olive oil, rosemary, grated garlic, and/or chopped onions.

Grass-fed and pasture-raised meats have different fat profiles than grain-fed meats. They have more anti-inflammatory omega-3 fats but less total fat, so they tend to dry out more easily. Because intramuscular fat acts like an insulator, these naturally lean meats cook more quickly than grain-fed meats of similar size. If you can, buy cuts that come with an exterior layer of fat to ensure that the meat won't dry out during cooking.

Season meat ahead and allow enough time for it to penetrate throughout, a minimum of 8 hours before you cook it and ideally 24 to 48 hours in advance. Use salt or a marinade containing salt, about ½ teaspoon per pound for boneless cuts and about ¾ teaspoon per pound for bone-in roasts. Like fish and poultry, meat should be at room temperature before you cook it, so take it out of the fridge an hour or so (depending on the side of the meat) in advance.

Long, slow cooking gives connective tissues the chance to break down. It melts and moistens the meat while it cooks, rendering it succulent and fall-apart tender. For cuts of meat other than ground meat and tender pieces like steak that cook quickly, brown the meat on the stove top before transferring it to the oven. Roast it in dry heat with fat but no liquid, or braise it in moist heat with water, bone broth, or wine (enough to fill the roasting pan with a couple of inches of liquid). Either way, cook meat at a low temperature (250 to 300°F) and determine doneness by internal temperature, not cooking time (although it's good to have an estimate of cooking time, so you'll know when to start checking the temperature).

Internal Temperatures of Meats and Poultry

In most cases, the less you cook meat, the healthier and more tender it is. Chicken should always be fully cooked, but duck, lamb, pork, beef, buffalo, and venison don't need to be. At temperatures above 170°F, proteins in meat change shape and create new bonds between molecules that make meat tough. Cooking meat too much also creates toxic compounds like PAHs and HCAs, destroys nutrients like vitamins and antioxidants, and damages omega-3 fats.

For perfectly done meats, cook them until they reach these internal temperatures:

- Beef, buffalo, lamb, and venison: 115 to 120°F (rare) or 125 to 130°F (medium rare)
- Pork: 140 to 145°F (trace of pink)
- Duck breast: 145 to 150°F (medium rare)
- Chicken and all other poultry: 165 to 170°F (thoroughly cooked)

Monitoring the internal temperature of meats is the best way to make sure that they won't be undercooked or overcooked. I recommend using an oven-safe mercury thermometer (plastic-free, less expensive, and more accurate than electric thermometers). Place roasts in the very center of your oven and, to ensure even heating, rotate them 180 degrees after cooking an hour (for smaller roasts) or two hours (for larger roasts). When you open the oven to rotate the roasting pan, stick the thermometer into the thickest part of the meat so that it will be easily visible. Monitor the temperature from time to time, more frequently the closer it gets to the target temperature.

After the meat is perfectly cooked, transfer it to a warm serving plate. Cover loosely (tented aluminum foil works well) and allow it to rest for at least ten minutes in a spot that's slightly warmer than room temperature. If your roast is large, you may want to let it rest for twenty minutes or more. Letting meats rest before you cut them allows the juices to be retained, which keeps the meat moist. In some cases, it also allows the meat to finish cooking, as the internal temperature will continue to rise in the first 10 minutes after you remove it from the heat.

If you're cooking meat on the stove top, don't cut into it to evaluate how done it is. Use your senses of sight, smell, and touch instead. You can learn how to associate texture with doneness by practicing on your hand. First find the muscle at the base of one of your thumbs, below the knuckle. Gently touch the tip of that thumb to the tip of the index finger on the same hand (without squeezing). With your other hand, feel how firm your thumb muscle is. That's close to how a rare steak would feel. If you touch the tip of your thumb to the tip of your middle finger, that's about medium-rare. Use your ring finger for medium and your pinky for medium-well. Once you learn the textures, you can use clean fingers or a utensil to gently press into meats on the stove top to estimate how done they are.

The techniques for making a pan sauce and saving rendered fat that I described for poultry can also be used with meats like beef, lamb, pork, and venison. See recipe: Moroccan Sliders With Lemon Yogurt Sauce.

Recipes

Morning Detox Smoothie

Making a smoothie for breakfast each morning is a quick and easy way to start the day right: with protein, healthy fat, and fiber. You can make it in just a minute or two, and it's a good way to get ground flaxseeds into your diet. Because every meal should contain a green vegetable, I like to throw in a handful of organic baby spinach, which purées nicely, thanks to its tender texture. You can use any leafy green you like or simply add a scoop of unsweetened green powder (go to www.prediabetesdetox.com for recommendations).

All berries have antioxidant and anti-inflammatory activity in the body, but I chose blackberries for this recipe because they can reverse pesticide-inflicted damage. If you don't have blackberries, you can use raspberries or blueberries, as long as they're organic. Frozen berries give the smoothie an icy cold quality and are available year-round.

This recipe calls for yogurt, but you can make a dairy-free smoothie by substituting a half cup of presoaked raw almonds, a quarter cup of raw almond butter, or two scoops of protein powder (see chapter 4 for more information about protein powders or visit www.pre diabetesdetox.com).

1 cup filtered water

½ cup organic frozen blackberries

½ cup organic baby spinach, chopped

½ cup organic whole-milk yogurt

2 tablespoons freshly ground flaxseeds

Pinch of ground cinnamon or ½ teaspoon freshly grated ginger

Add all of all of the ingredients to a blender and blend until smooth. Drink the smoothie immediately.

Makes 2 cups

Artichoke Olive Tapenade

This simple starter takes just minutes to throw together with a food processor. You can make it without a food processor if you finely chop the ingredients, but it won't come together as quickly and the texture will not be quite as fine.

This recipe doesn't call for salt, because the olives, anchovies, and Parmesan are naturally salty. For a dairy-free version, omit the cheese. If your lemon isn't organic, omit the zest. If you're not a fan of anchovies, add them anyway. They won't give the tapenade a fishy flavor, just a salty and savory taste. No one will ever guess they're in there.

Serve this tapenade with cucumber rounds as a starter or as a condiment with fish, poultry, or meat.

- 1 (12-ounce) package frozen artichoke hearts, thawed and drained
- ½ cup pitted and roughly chopped green olives
- ¼ cup freshly grated Parmesan cheese (optional)
- ¼ cup cold-pressed extra-virgin olive oil
- 3 anchovy fillets
- 1 to 2 cloves garlic, roughly chopped
- Freshly ground pepper
- 1 organic lemon, zested and juiced

Add the artichokes, olives, cheese, oil, anchovies, garlic, pepper, lemon zest, and 2 tablespoons of lemon juice to a food processor. Pulse until everything is finely chopped.

Taste the tapenade and add more lemon juice or pepper if needed.

Serve the tapenade immediately or transfer it to an airtight container and store in the fridge for up to three days.

Makes about 2 cups

Roasted Beet Salad

This salad makes a simple starter or side dish and can be served warm or at room temperature. If you want to serve it as a main course, add some protein, such as a soft- or hard-boiled egg, peeled and quartered.

Because vegetables are best roasted at high temperatures (400°F), this recipe calls for ghee, a stable saturated fat. You can also use coconut oil or rendered chicken or duck fat. If you use coconut oil, your finished dish will have a different flavor.

> 2 large or 3 medium beets, root and stem ends trimmed, cut into wedges of similar size
>
> 1 tablespoon ghee
>
> Sea salt
>
> Freshly ground pepper
>
> 1 tablespoon aged balsamic vinegar
>
> 1 tablespoon cold-pressed extra-virgin olive oil
>
> ½ cup pitted Kalamata or other olives, roughly chopped
>
> ½ cup chopped walnuts
>
> Crumbled goat cheese (optional)

Preheat the oven to 400°F.

Melt the ghee in a stainless-steel or glass mixing bowl set over a pan containing an inch or two of gently simmering water (the water should not be touching the bowl). Remove the bowl from the heat as soon as the ghee has melted. Toss the beets in the melted ghee until they are evenly coated.

Arrange the beets on a baking sheet without crowding them, sprinkle them with salt and pepper, and roast them until they are tender and lightly browned, 30 to 60 minutes depending on the size of your wedges.

In a mixing bowl, whisk together the vinegar and oil. Stir in the beets, olives, and walnuts until thoroughly coated with the vinaigrette. Transfer to a serving plate and garnish with goat cheese just before serving.

> Makes about 2 cups

Making Your Own Ghee

Ghee is pure butter fat, without the milk solids. It's a good choice for high-temperature cooking. Use ghee to replace inflammatory oils in any recipe or to replace healthy but fragile olive oil in dishes that call for more than gentle cooking.

It's easy to make your own ghee, and there's only one ingredient: a pound of unsalted butter. Use the best quality butter you can find and warm it in a saucepan over medium-low heat. After it melts and starts simmering, turn the heat down to low. Allow the butter to cook gently, uncovered, until it turns clear, about 20 minutes. If the curds that form at the bottom of the pan begin to brown, lower the heat.

Allow the ghee to cool slightly, then strain it through a fine mesh strainer lined with cheesecloth into a clean glass jar. Close the jar with a tight-fitting lid, and store the ghee at room temperature. It will last for a very long time.

Cauliflower with Walnut Pesto

Pesto is really just a paste, and it can be made of many different things. Often pesto includes fresh herbs, garlic, some sort of nut, and something salty, like grated Parmesan cheese, olives, or anchovies. This version calls for basil, but you can use any fresh herb or mixture of herbs that you like. I used walnuts because they are an exceptionally good source of healthy omega-3 fats. If you prefer dairy-free pesto, opt for olives or anchovies instead of Parmesan.

Pesto is one of the most versatile condiments. Slather it on slices of fresh tomatoes and mozzarella cheese for a simple starter. Toss it with cooked vegetables like artichokes, asparagus, broccoli, baby peas, eggplant, leafy green vegetables, string beans, summer squash, or zucchini for a flavorful side dish. Thin it out with more olive oil and a dash of red wine vinegar to make pesto vinaigrette. Serve it as a dip for raw vegetables or as a condiment with fish, poultry, or meat. This recipe yields about a cup of pesto, but you'll only need ¼ cup to finish the dish. Store the leftover pesto in an airtight container in the fridge for up to a week or in the freezer for several months.

In this recipe, you can substitute rendered chicken or duck fat for the ghee.

> 1 bunch fresh basil (about 3 cups packed leaves)
>
> ⅓ cup grated Parmesan cheese
>
> ⅔ cup raw walnuts
>
> 2 cloves garlic, smashed and chopped
>
> ½ cup cold-pressed extra-virgin olive oil
>
> ¼ teaspoon sea salt
>
> Freshly ground pepper to taste
>
> 1 tablespoon ghee
>
> 1 head of cauliflower, finely chopped

Add the basil, Parmesan, walnuts, garlic, oil, salt, and pepper to a food processor or blender and purée until smooth. Taste the mixture and adjust the seasoning if necessary.

Heat the ghee in a large skillet over medium heat. Add the cauliflower, season with salt and pepper, and cook until tender and lightly browned, stirring occasionally, about 10 minutes. If the cauliflower starts to stick to the pan before it starts to brown, add a bit more ghee. If the cauliflower is soft but not brown, increase the heat to medium-high and continue cooking until it develops some color. (Up to this point, without the pesto, this is how I prepare cauliflower couscous.) Turn off the heat. Stir in ¼ cup of pesto and toss until the cauliflower is thoroughly coated. Serve immediately.

Makes 2 to 3 cups, depending on the size of your cauliflower

Brussels Sprout Sauté

Brussel sprouts are bite-sized cabbages that grow on a stalk. When you slow-cook them, they develop a naturally sweet and nutty flavor. Sautéed until caramelized and golden brown, these brussels sprouts even leave skeptics asking for more.

Brussels sprouts can be cut by hand with a sharp knife, but a food processor makes this task a snap. I always make as much as my largest skillet will hold to be sure to have leftovers.

A word on adding salt: Generally wait until the sprouts have caramelized, as adding salt will draw out water and can keep the sprouts from browning. If they are starting to stick to the pan before browning, however, it can be helpful to add a little salt to draw out some moisture.

You can substitute rendered chicken or duck fat for the ghee in this recipe.

> 1 tablespoon ghee
>
> 1 pound fresh brussels sprouts, washed, trimmed, and thinly sliced
>
> Sea salt
>
> Freshly ground pepper
>
> Pinch of freshly grated nutmeg
>
> Juice of ½ fresh lemon
>
> 2 to 3 tablespoons grass-fed or organic heavy cream

Warm the ghee in a large skillet over medium heat. Add the brussels sprouts and sauté, stirring occasionally, until golden brown and caramelized, about 20 minutes. If they start to stick, stir in a small amount of salt.

When the brussels sprouts are tender and browned, season with salt, pepper and nutmeg. Stir in half of the lemon juice and just enough cream to coat the leaves and distribute the seasoning evenly. Taste and adjust the seasoning if necessary. Serve immediately.

Makes about 3 cups

Everyday Salad with Homemade Vinaigrette

Vinaigrettes are easy to whip up on the spot, and I like making them to order, so I can tailor them to best complement the rest of the meal. I usually have several kinds of vinegar on hand, and simply substituting one for another can dramatically transform the finished flavor. Sometimes I substitute fresh citrus juice for the vinegar. If you prefer to keep a jar of vinaigrette in the fridge, increase the ingredients listed below, add them to a clean glass jar with a tight-fitting lid, and shake it up each time you use it.

1 tablespoon red wine vinegar

1 clove garlic, grated

Sea salt

1 teaspoon Dijon-style mustard or ½ teaspoon ground mustard seed

Freshly ground pepper

3 tablespoons cold-pressed extra-virgin olive oil

6 cups salad greens

¼ small red onion, cut into very thin slices

½ red bell pepper, cut into very thin slices

½ cup raw walnuts

Add the vinegar, garlic, and a small pinch of salt to the bottom of your largest bowl and set it aside for a few minutes to allow the garlic to soften and the salt to dissolve. Whisk in the mustard and ground pepper. Stream in the oil and continue whisking until it becomes a smooth and homogeneous mixture. Taste and adjust the seasoning if necessary.

Add the onion, red pepper, and walnuts to the bowl, and place your salad greens on top. Toss all of the ingredients together and serve the salad immediately, or set the bowl aside until you're ready to eat it. Toss it at the last moment to prevent crispy greens from getting soggy.

Makes about 7 cups

Vinaigrette Variations:

To make balsamic vinaigrette, substitute balsamic vinegar for the red wine vinegar.

To make citrus vinaigrette, add the zest of a lemon or orange and substitute freshly squeezed lemon juice for the vinegar.

To make raspberry vinaigrette, add ¼ cup of frozen raspberries, thawed and mashed, with their juices.

To make green vinaigrette, add fresh herbs and minced shallot.

For a creamy vinaigrette, add a spoonful of Greek or strained yogurt.

Kale with Anchovies, Lemon, and Garlic

If you don't have kale, you can use any green leafy vegetable in this dish. Anchovies add a savory flavor, not a fishy one, so add them even if you think you don't like them (especially if you don't like them because you've probably never had them like this before). If your anchovies are packed in salt, soak them in water to remove excess salt before you use them.

If you don't have ghee, you can use butter or olive oil, but lower the heat to medium-low and extend the cooking time.

> 2 tablespoons ghee
>
> 5 anchovy fillets
>
> Pinch of cayenne
>
> 1 bunch kale, stemmed, leaves cut into 1-inch strips
>
> 1 organic lemon
>
> 2 cloves garlic

Warm the ghee in a large skillet over medium heat. Add the anchovies and cook them for a few minutes until they break down. Stir in the cayenne.

Add the kale, in batches if necessary, and toss it with the fat in the bottom of the skillet. Cover the pan and cook until the leaves are wilted and tender, stirring occasionally, about 5 minutes.

After you turn off the heat, use a grater to zest the lemon and grate the garlic directly into the skillet. Cut the lemon in half and add a dash of juice. Toss the kale to thoroughly incorporate the lemon and garlic.

Taste and adjust the seasoning if necessary, adding more lemon juice or a pinch of sea salt (although the anchovies will probably make it salty enough). Serve immediately.

> Makes about 2 cups

Bone Broth

Broth made from bones has been consumed as both food and medicine since ancient times. Both delicious and nutritious, rich in minerals and glistening with fat droplets, bone broth has been called "liquid gold." Bone broth contains amino acids like glycine; minerals like calcium, magnesium, potassium, and phosphorus; and glycosaminoglycans (building blocks for connective tissues like bones, blood vessels, and skin). These nutrients are especially well absorbed, and gelatin from the bones acts as a natural digestive aid. Bone broth can be consumed as is or used as a healthy base for soups, stews, and sauces.

Like all things, the quality of the finished product can only be as good as the quality of the ingredients. Use bones from animals raised on pasture, fed their natural diet, and never exposed to hormones, antibiotics, pesticides, or other chemicals.

This recipe calls for turkey bones, but you can use bones from any wild, grass-fed, or pasture-raised animal (chicken, duck, beef, lamb, or pork). The bones can be fresh from your butcher; they can come from meat you've already cooked; or you can use fresh chicken feet or wings, which are inexpensive and widely available. It's best to use bones with some meat still attached if you can, as they make the most flavorful and nutritious broths. Bones attached to joints are best, for they contain the most connective tissue.

To facilitate the transfer of nutrients into the broth, the bones should have some marrow exposed. If you have sharp kitchen shears or a sharp cleaver, you can chop up poultry bones yourself. If you're not comfortable doing this or if you don't have a cleaver, ask your butcher to chop them for you. If you're using thicker bones (like those from beef, lamb, or pork), power tools will be required to cut them, and you should definitely ask your butcher to do it for you. The bones don't need to end up in tiny pieces, but they do need to fit into your cooking pot.

Broths made with poultry bones, like this one, should be simmered slowly for at least 6 hours. Broths made from fish bones or crab, lobster, or shrimp shells should be simmered slowly for only 2 hours. Broths made from thicker bones should be simmered slowly for at least 24 hours (a slow cooker works well), and the vegetables should be added in the last few hours of cooking.

This recipe doesn't call for much salt. You can add more later, depending on what you plan to use the broth for. I recommend adding a little vinegar to maximize the release of minerals and gelatin from the bones as the broth simmers. The measurements for bones and vegetables in this recipe aren't very specific, because you can make bone broth from varying amounts of ingredients and in pots of varying sizes. Only bones and water are required, but beans add body, and vegetables and aromatics like bay leaves add flavor. As a general rule, fill your stockpot at least half full of bones, add any other ingredients you like, leaving at least 3 inches of room at the top; then cover everything with water, leaving an inch or so of room at the top, and add a dash of vinegar. If you don't have enough bones to fill a pot at least halfway full, store them in the freezer until you do. You can also freeze vegetable scraps like leek tops and celery ends until you're ready to make bone broth.

If you have limited storage space, you can reduce the broth at a boil after you remove the solids, so you're left with less volume but more concentrated flavor. You can add water later if you're using the broth as a base stock for other recipes. I also like to freeze some of the broth in an ice-cube tray to add to pan sauces or other dishes that need only small amounts of stock.

This recipe makes about 6 pints of broth using an 8-quart stockpot.

Several cups of meaty turkey carcass, with marrow exposed

Several cups of roughly chopped aromatic vegetables like celery, carrots, onions, or leeks

A head of garlic, cut in half horizontally

½ teaspoon sea salt

1 teaspoon whole peppercorns

1 fresh bay leaf or 2 to 3 dried bay leaves

1 or 2 dried chili peppers

½ cup dried beans (adzuki, kidney, or pinto), soaked for 8 to 24 hours

2 tablespoons apple cider vinegar per quart of water

Add everything to a large stockpot along with enough cold water to cover all the ingredients. Bring to a boil, and reduce to a low simmer. Cover and cook for 6 hours at a boil so gentle that just a few bubbles rise to the surface at a time. Skim off any foam that rises to the surface.

Once the bone broth has finished cooking, you can skim off some of the fat floating on top to use for high-temperature cooking. You also can leave the fat in to enrich the broth.

If you don't plan to use the broth right away, allow it to cool completely before putting in the fridge. An easy way to cool it down quickly is to remove as much of the solids as possible with a slotted spoon, then pour the slightly cooled broth through a fine mesh strainer into a second large pot, and portion it into clean glass jars with tight-fitting lids, allowing at least an inch of space at the top. I use a glass measuring cup with a pouring spout to transfer the broth to widemouthed pint-size canning jars, as they stand up well in the freezer (larger canning jars or less sturdy jars often crack). Once the broth has cooled to room temperature or after 2 hours, place the lids on the jars, transfer them to the fridge, and allow them to chill overnight (the broth should develop a gel-like consistency). The following day, transfer to the freezer any jars you don't plan to use in the near future. Leave the lids off, for the liquid will expand as it freezes, and you don't want the jars to burst (this is why you left an inch of space at the top). The following day, when the stock is completely frozen, screw on the lids.

Makes 6 pints or more

Medicinal Mushroom Soup

This soup is good for detox, but it's also good for colds and flu (shiitake and maitake mushrooms have been extensively studied for their positive effects on immunity). Puréeing part of the soup, then reincorporating it, gives this soup a thick and creamy texture. It's a good way to thicken soups without adding flour or potato starch, and it also keeps it dairy-free.

Find maitake mushrooms at your local farmers' market and possibly even your grocery store. If they're not in season, use another type of mushroom or add more shiitakes (avoid white button mushrooms, because their flavor is too mild for this soup). You'll only use the shiitake caps, so save the stems for your next batch of bone broth (see recipe).

This recipe calls for parsley because of its positive effects on blood sugar control, but you could use fresh thyme, rosemary, or oregano. If you don't have fresh herbs, use one teaspoon of dried herbs, but add them with the bone broth, instead of at the end of cooking, so they have time to rehydrate and flavor the dish. Grind or crush dried herbs before adding them, if you can.

    1 large portobello mushroom cap

    Cold-pressed extra-virgin olive oil

    Sea salt

    Freshly ground pepper

    2 leeks, halved lengthwise, cut into ¼-inch-thick slices, and thoroughly cleaned

    1½ cups shiitake mushroom caps, cut into ⅛-inch-thick slices

    1½ cups maitake mushrooms, cut into ⅛-inch-thick slices

    4 cups bone broth

    1 bay leaf

    2 garlic cloves

    2 tablespoons finely chopped fresh parsley

    Additional chopped fresh parsley for garnish

Preheat the broiler. Wipe the portobello cap clean with a damp cloth and place it gill-side up in a shallow baking dish. Drizzle it with oil and sprinkle it with salt and pepper. Broil the mushroom until it becomes tender and the gills start to crisp, about 7 minutes. Set it aside to cool slightly, then cut it into ½-inch dice, and reserve any juices.

Warm two tablespoons of oil in a soup pot over medium-low heat. Add the leeks, shiitakes, maitakes, and a pinch each of salt and pepper. Sauté the mixture until the mushrooms become soft and start to brown, about 10 minutes.

Stir in the bone broth, bay leaf, and diced portobello with any juices. Bring the mixture to a boil, reduce the heat to low, and simmer for thirty minutes. Turn off the heat and allow the soup to cool, uncovered, for thirty minutes.

Transfer about half of the soup to a blender or food processor and purée until smooth, working in batches if necessary. Return the puréed soup to the pot and stir until well incorporated.

Grate the garlic cloves into the soup and stir in the parsley. Taste and adjust the seasoning if necessary. To serve, gently reheat the soup over medium-low heat. Garnish with fresh parsley and serve immediately.

Makes about 6 cups

Thai Curry with Tempeh and Mixed Vegetables

There are several different kinds of curries, and they come from all over the world, including Thailand, India, Malaysia, and the Caribbean. Red curry pastes use ripe red chili peppers, and green curry pastes use green chili peppers. Green curry pastes are usually milder and less intense than the red varieties.

It's possible to make curry paste from scratch, but some of the ingredients (like fresh lemongrass, kefir lime, and galangal) aren't always readily available. If you want to make your own, you can find a recipe at www.prediabetesdetox.com. Fortunately, it's no longer difficult to find good-quality prepared curry pastes full of anti-inflammatory, detox-supportive, blood sugar–lowering spices. Ingredients like ginger, garlic, and salt act as natural antimicrobial agents, making added preservatives unnecessary. Use a fresh curry paste if you can find it. If you want to make your own, you can find a recipe at www. prediabetesdetox.com.

Once you have curry paste and coconut milk, this dish is a snap. It's also incredibly versatile, as you can use any protein and vegetables you like. Instead of tempeh, try salmon, sablefish, shrimp, mussels, chicken, duck, beef, or lamb. Add more curry paste for a stronger and spicier flavor or less for a more mild dish. If you have a food processor, use it to make quick work of finely chopping the cauliflower.

4 tablespoons coconut oil

1 small head cauliflower, finely chopped

8 ounces tempeh, cut into 1-inch cubes

1 small onion, halved and cut into ½-inch-thick slices

8 cups of vegetables, like leafy greens, broccoli, and mushrooms, cut into bite-sized pieces

1 to 2 tablespoons panang curry paste or other curry paste

14 ounces coconut milk

2 teaspoons fish sauce

Heat the oil in two large skillets (two tablespoons of oil per pan) over medium heat. To one skillet, add the cauliflower and season it with salt and pepper. Cook, stirring occasionally, until soft and starting to brown, about 15 minutes.

Add the tempeh to the other skillet. Cook until browned on all sides, turning them as needed. Add the onion and mixed vegetables. Continue cooking until these start to soften, 5 to 10 minutes, depending on the size and density of vegetables. Push the vegetables toward the sides of the skillet, making space in the middle. Add the curry paste to the empty spot and sauté until it softens and becomes aromatic. Stir the curry paste into the vegetables until evenly distributed. Stir in the coconut milk and continue cooking until the vegetables are tender and fully cooked. Turn off the heat and stir in 1 teaspoon of fish sauce. Taste for seasoning. Add an additional teaspoon of fish sauce if you prefer a saltier and more savory flavor.

To serve this dish, arrange a bed of the sautéed cauliflower on a serving plate and spoon the tempeh, vegetables, and curry sauce over the top.

Makes 4 main course servings

Blackened Salmon

This dish is blackened with spices. It's a healthy alternative to charring meats, which creates cancer-causing compounds. The spice rub is versatile, and once you have it ready, you can make this dish in minutes. Use what's leftover on sablefish, haddock, Atlantic pollock, tempeh, poultry, or pork.

I like to grind whole spices just before using them to ensure the freshest flavors and the most medicinal benefits. In this dish, I used smoked paprika and smoked sea salt to give a grilled flavor. (Smoking chili peppers and sea salt doesn't create the same carcinogens as smoking meat and fish.) If you don't have dried thyme, you can use dried oregano or rosemary. If you don't have dried chipotle, you can use cayenne, red pepper flakes, or any other dried chili pepper. I like to save lime zest whenever I'm juicing a lime, so I often have it on hand. I add it to loose-leaf tea or spice rubs like this one. If you don't have any, you can use fresh lime or lemon zest. If you don't have mixed peppercorns, you can use black peppercorns.

- 1 dried chipotle chili pepper, stem removed and cut into pieces with sharp kitchen shears
- 1 tablespoon mixed peppercorns
- 1 tablespoon dried thyme leaves
- 1 tablespoon smoked paprika
- 1 tablespoon smoked sea salt or other sea salt
- 1 teaspoon cumin seeds or 1 teaspoon ground cumin
- 1 teaspoon dried organic lime zest
- 1 pound wild salmon fillets, cut into 4 even portions, at room temperature
- 1 tablespoon ghee or coconut oil
- Chopped fresh cilantro or parsley to garnish
- Whole-milk Greek yogurt to garnish (optional)
- Fresh lemon or lime wedges for serving

Put the chipotle, peppercorns, thyme, paprika, salt, cumin, and lime zest into a clean electric grinder (or mortar and pestle) and grind until smooth.

Place a tablespoon or two of the mixture on a large plate and gently swirl it around to distribute the seasoning evenly. Place the salmon fillets, skin side up, onto the plate. Flip the salmon onto another plate and rub the mixture into the seasoned side to coat thoroughly.

Heat the ghee in a large skillet over medium heat until hot. Add the salmon, seasoned side down. Cook the fish about 4 to 5 minutes, until it lifts easily away from the skillet.

Flip the salmon, cover the pan, and turn off the heat. Finish cooking the fish with residual heat, about 5 to 7 minutes more, depending on the size and thickness of the fish.

Toss a salad while you wait for the salmon to finish cooking. Garnish the fish with fresh cilantro or parsley, top each piece with a dollop of yogurt if you wish, and serve immediately with fresh lemon or lime wedges.

Makes 4 main course servings

Braised Chicken Legs with Olives and Lemon

This one-pot dish is delicious and easy to make. You start this dish on the stove top and then finish it off in the oven. While it's baking, you're free to make a side dish or two. I like to serve the chicken legs on a bed of sautéed winter greens or over an artichoke and white bean purée with the sauce spooned over the top.

This recipe calls for two chicken legs (thigh and drumstick), but I like to use duck legs whenever I have them. It serves two to four people, depending on how large the legs are and what you're serving on the side. If you have a crowd to feed, use a whole chicken, cut into pieces of similar size, and double the amount of other ingredients.

Preserved lemons give this dish a pleasingly complex flavor. Most people advise using only the peel, but I use the whole lemon after I remove the seeds. Taste the fruit, and if you think it tastes good, use the whole lemon. If you don't care for the fruit, discard it, and add only the peel. It's okay if it tastes a little bit salty, as you won't need to add additional salt. If you think it's *too* salty, rinse it well or soak it in water for a few minutes before you cut into it. You can find preserved lemons packed in jars in well-stocked grocery stores, buy them online, or learn to make them yourself. Preserving lemons takes only two ingredients (lemons and salt), and you can find an easy recipe at www.prediabetesdetox.com.

If you don't have preserved lemon, use the zest of an organic lemon and some of the juice, but add these along with the garlic at the end of cooking, so they don't turn bitter. If you don't have rendered chicken or duck fat, you can use ghee. Don't use a liquid oil, because a saturated fat is needed to withstand the temperature required to brown the chicken.

- 1 tablespoon rendered chicken or duck fat
- 2 skin-on, bone-in chicken legs (thigh plus drumstick) at room temperature, seasoned with sea salt 24 to 48 hours in advance
- 1 small onion, halved and cut into ⅛-inch-thick slices
- 1 preserved lemon, quartered, seeded, and cut into ⅛-inch-thick slices

1 cup of green olives, pitted

¼ teaspoon ground cinnamon

½ teaspoon ground turmeric

½ teaspoon ground cumin

½ teaspoon smoked paprika or regular paprika

½ to 1 teaspoon freshly grated ginger

1 cup bone broth

2 cloves garlic

Preheat the oven to 300°F.

Warm the fat in a deep ovenproof skillet, or a shallow Dutch oven large enough to accommodate the chicken legs comfortably, over medium heat until hot. Brown the chicken legs on both sides. Transfer to a plate.

Add the onion to the pan and cook until soft and starting to brown, about five minutes. Stir in the lemon, olives, cinnamon, turmeric, cumin, paprika, ginger, and bone broth.

Place the chicken legs skin side up on top of the other ingredients. Cover and bake in the oven for an hour or more, until the joints are loose, the meat is tender, and the internal temperature registers at least 170°F. If you prefer a crispy skin, place it under the broiler, uncovered, for a couple of minutes at the end.

Transfer the chicken legs to a serving plate. Grate the garlic cloves directly into the sauce left in the pan. Stir to incorporate the garlic thoroughly. Spoon the sauce over the top and serve immediately.

Makes 2 to 4 main course servings, depending on the size of your chicken legs

Moroccan Sliders with Lemon Yogurt Sauce

These two-bite burgers are bursting with flavor, thanks to a winning combination of savory lamb, aromatics like fresh cilantro, ginger, and garlic, and ground spices like cinnamon and turmeric. If you don't have turmeric, buy it. If you're missing another spice or two, don't sweat it. Your variation will likely be tasty too.

I used pine nuts in this recipe, but you can use any raw nuts you like (pistachios also go well with lamb). I also used a food processor to grind up some of the ingredients, but you could use a mortar and pestle. If you do, finely chop everything first.

Serve these sliders with a big salad instead of a bun. As an alternative to patties, the meat mixture can be molded around stainless-steel or wooden skewers that have been soaked in water (to prevent them from catching fire). Either way, you can prepare the mixture in advance and cook them on demand. The lemon yogurt sauce can be made ahead as well, and it couldn't be more simple (it's just lemon and yogurt). Be sure that your lemon is organic if you're using the zest.

½ cup raw pine nuts

½ cup (packed) fresh cilantro leaves and stems

2 or 3 garlic cloves, smashed and coarsely chopped

2 or 3 teaspoons fresh grated ginger

½ cup roughly chopped onion

¼ teaspoon sea salt

½ teaspoon ground turmeric

¼ teaspoon black pepper

½ teaspoon ground coriander

¼ teaspoon ground cumin

¼ teaspoon ground cinnamon

¼ teaspoon ground allspice

Pinch of ground cardamom

Pinch or more of cayenne pepper

1½ pounds ground grass-fed lamb

Ghee or rendered animal fat, for cooking

Lemon Yogurt Sauce

1 organic lemon, zest and juice

½ cup whole-milk Greek or strained yogurt

Toast the pine nuts in a dry skillet over low heat, until aromatic and just starting to brown. Set them aside to cool.

Put the pine nuts with the cilantro, garlic, ginger, onion, and salt into a food processor and pulse until finely chopped. Transfer the mixture to a large mixing bowl. Stir in the turmeric, peppers, coriander, cumin, cinnamon, allspice, cardamom, and cayenne until well combined.

Add the ground lamb to the bowl and, using impeccably clean hands, combine all the ingredients. Do not overwork the meat, but make sure that everything is evenly incorporated.

Heat a small amount of fat in a skillet over medium heat. (You won't need much, because the lamb will release a lot of fat.) Make a small test patty, cook it through on both sides, and taste it for seasoning. If necessary, adjust the seasoning and cook another test patty. Once you're happy with the flavor, form the rest of the lamb mixture into twelve balls, then gently flatten them into patties. (The sliders can be prepared ahead up to this point and stored in an airtight container in the fridge or freezer.)

Heat a small amount of fat in a large skillet over medium heat (if you've just made a test patty, you likely won't need any more fat). Cook the patties until well browned, about five minutes on each side. Serve the lamb sliders with the lemon yogurt sauce (recipe follows). If you have winter greens on hand, transfer the sliders from the pan to a covered dish to keep them warm while you quickly cook the greens, covered, in the pan juices. Otherwise serve the sliders with a big green salad.

To make the sauce: Stir all of the lemon zest and a teaspoon of the juice into the yogurt. Taste it and add more juice if desired. You can add a pinch of sea salt and ground peppercorn if you wish, but it doesn't really need it, and left unseasoned, any leftover sauce makes an excellent dip for fresh strawberries.

Makes 12 sliders (6 main course servings or 12 appetizer servings)

Dark Chocolate Clusters

These two-bite clusters are full of antioxidants, healthy fats, and protein, and they're easy to make. They'll only taste as good as the chocolate you use, so pick one of good quality.

You can use small paper baking cups (like those used for mini-muffins) or a silicone mold to make these clusters. If you use paper cups with a diameter of 1¼ to 1½ inches or a mold with 1¼-inch squares, this recipe will yield 21 clusters. You can eat three of these clusters per day, because you're allowed 1 ounce of dark chocolate per day and this recipe uses 7 ounces of chocolate. If you use a different-size mold, or if you end up with a different number of clusters, remember that your daily intake should be limited to one-seventh of the total yield.

> 7 ounces 85 percent dark chocolate
>
> 1 cup unsweetened coconut flakes
>
> 1 cup raw walnut pieces

Place the dark chocolate in a large glass or stainless-steel mixing bowl over a pan of gently simmering water. The water should not be touching the bowl. As soon as the chocolate has just melted, turn off the heat and transfer the bowl to a heat-proof surface like a wooden cutting board or a kitchen towel folded in quarters. Monitor the chocolate closely and do *not* overheat the chocolate.

Stir in the coconut and walnuts until they are thoroughly coated with chocolate.

Portion the mixture into small paper baking cups or a silicone mold and place inside the fridge for at least 2 hours. Once the clusters have set, unmold them if you're using a mold. If you're using paper cups, you can leave them in the cups if you wish. Transfer the clusters to a covered glass container and store in the fridge.

Before serving, allow them to come to room temperature.

> Makes 21 clusters

References

Abou-Donia, M. B., E. M. El-Masry, A. A. Abdel-Rahman, R. E. McLendon, and S. S. Schiffman. 2008. "Splenda Alters Gut Microflora and Increases Intestinal P-Glycoprotein and Cytochrome P-450 in Male Rats." *Journal of Toxicology and Environmental Health* 71(21): 1415–29.

Akerstedt, T., B. Arnetz, G. Ficca, L. E. Paulsson, and A. Kallner. 1999. "A 50-Hz Electromagnetic Field Impairs Sleep." *Journal of Sleep Research* 8 (1): 77–81.

Allport, S. 2006. *The Queen of Fats: Why Omega-3s Were Removed fro the Western Diet and What We Can Do to Replace Them.* Berkeley: University of California Press.

Alonso-Magdalena, P., A. B. Ropero, S. Soriano, I. Quesada, and A. Nadal. 2010. "Bisphenol-A: A New Diabetogenic Factor?" *Hormones* (Athens) 9 (2): 118–26.

Alonso-Magdalena, P., I. Quesada, and A. Nadal. 2011. "Endocrine Disruptors in the Etiology of Type 2 Diabetes Mellitus." *Nature Reviews. Endocrinology* 7 (6): 346–53.

Angelieri, C. T., C. R. Barros, A. Siqueira-Catani, and S. R. Ferreira. 2012. "Trans-Fatty Acid Intake Is Associated with Insulin Sensitivity but Independently of Inflammation." *Brazilian Journal of Medical and Biological Research* 45 (7): 625–31.

Angima, S. 2010. "Toxic Heavy Metals in Farm Soil." *Small Farms* V (3). http://smallfarms.oregonstate.edu/sfn/su10toxicmetals.

ATSDR (Agency for Toxic Substances and Disease Registry). 2008. "Cadmium Toxicity: What Is the Biological Fate of Cadmium in the Body?" Case Study in Environmental Medicine, Centers for Disease Control and Prevention, Atlanta. http://www.atsdr.cdc.gov/csem/csem .asp?csem=6&po=9.

Ballali, S., and F. Lanciai. 2011. "Functional Food and Diabetes: A Natural Way in Diabetes Prevention?" *International Journal of Food Sciences and Nutrition* 63 (Suppl 1): 51–61.

Barnard, R. J., E. J. Ugianskis, D. A. Martin, and S. B. Inkeles. 1992. "Role of Diet and Exercise in the Management of Hyperinsulinemia and Associated Atherosclerotic Risk Factors." *American Journal of Cardiology* 69 (5): 440–44.

Barriocanal, L. A., M. Palacios, G. Benitez, S. Benitez, J. T. Jimenez, N. Jimenez, and V. Rojas. 2008. "Apparent Lack of Pharmacological Effect of Steviol Glycosides Used as Sweeteners in Humans. A Pilot Study of Repeated Exposures in Some Normotensive and Hypotensive Individuals and in Type 1 and Type 2 Diabetics." *Regulatory Toxicology and Pharmacology* 51 (1): 37–41.

Beever, R. 2010. "The Effects of Repeated Thermal Therapy on Quality of Life in Patients with Type 2 Diabetes Mellitus." *Journal of Alternative and Complementary Medicine* 16 (6): 677–81.

Bender, N. K., M. A. Kraynak, E. Chiquette, W. D. Linn, G. M. Clark, and H. I. Bussey. 1998. "Effects of Marine Fish Oils on the Anticoagulation Status of Patients Receiving Chronic Warfarin Therapy." *Journal of Thrombosis and Thrombolysis* 5 (3): 257–61.

Boberg, J., S. Metzdorff, R. Wortziger, M. Axelstad, L. Brokken, A. M. Vinggaard, M. Dalgaard, and C Nellemann. 2008. "Impact of Diisobutyl Phthalate and Other PPAR Agonists on Steroidogenesis and Plasma Insulin and Leptin Levels in Fetal Rats." *Toxicology* 250 (2–3): 75–81.

Bolkent, S., R. Yanardag, O. Ozsoy-Sacan, and O. Karabulut-Bulan. 2004. "Effects of Parsley (Petroselinum Crispum) on the Liver of Diabetic Rats: A Morphological and Biochemical Study." *Phytotherapy Research* 18 (12): 996–99.

Boonjaraspinyo, S., T. Boonmars, C. Aromdee, A. Puapairoj, and Z. Wu. 2011. "Indirect Effect of a Turmeric Diet: Enhanced Bile Duct Proliferation in Syrian Hamsters with a Combination of Partial Obstruction by Opisthorchis Viverrini Infection and Inflammation by N-Nitrosodimethylamine Administration." *Parasitology Research* 108 (1): 7–14.

Bourre, J. M. 2005. "Where to Find Omega-3 Fatty Acids and How Feeding Animals with Diet Enriched in Omega-3 Fatty Acids to Increase Nutritional Value of Derived Products for Human: What Is Actually Useful?" *Journal of Nutrition, Health, and Aging* 9 (4): 232–42.

Bradley, R., K. J. Sherman, S. Catz, C. Calabrese, E. B. Oberg, L. Jordan, L. Grothaus, and D. Cherkin. 2012. "Adjunctive Naturopathic Care for Type 2 Diabetes: Patient-Reported and Clinical Outcomes After One Year." *BMC Complementary and Alternative Medicine* 12 (1): 44.

Burgomaster, K. A., S. C. Hughes, G. J. Heigenhauser, S. N. Bradwell, and M. J. Gibala. 2005. "Six Sessions of Sprint Interval Training Increases Muscle Oxidative Potential and Cycle Endurance Capacity in Humans." *Journal of Applied Physiology* 98 (6): 1985–90.

Cancer Prevention Coalition. 2003. "Carcinogens at Home." http://www .preventcancer.com/consumers/household/carcinogens_home.htm.

Casals-Casas, C., and B. Desvergne. 2011. "Endocrine Disruptors: from Endocrine to Metabolic Disruption." *Annual Review of Physiology* 73: 135–62.

CDC (Centers for Disease Control and Prevention). 2013. "Fourth National Report on Human Exposure to Environmental Chemicals, Updated Tables." US Department of Health and Human Services. http://www .cdc.gov/exposurereport.

CFS (Center for Food Safety). 2013. "GE Foods." http://www.centerforfood safety.org/issues/309/ge-fish/issues/311/ge-foods.

Chai, R. S., Y. F. Niu, L. Q. Zhu, H. Wang, and Y. S. Zhang. 2011. "Effects of Elevated CO2 Concentration on the Quality of Agricultural Products: A Review." Article in Chinese. *Ying Yong Sheng Tai Xue Bao* 22 (10): 2765–75.

Chan, Y. S., L. N. Cheng, J. H. Wu, E. Chan, Y. W. Kwan, S. M. Lee, G. P. Leung, P. H. Yu, and S. W. Chan. 2011. "A Review of the Pharmacological Effects of Arctium Lappa (Burdock)." *Inflammopharmacology* 19 (5): 245–54.

Chandalia M., A. Garg, D. Lutjohann, K. von Bergmann, S. M. Grundy, and L. J. Brinkley. 2000. "Beneficial Effects of High Dietary Fiber Intake in Patients with Type 2 Diabetes Mellitus." *New England Journal of Medicine* 342 (19): 1392–98.

Chang, J. C., M. C. Wu, I. M. Liu, and J. T. Cheng. 2005. "Increase of Insulin Sensitivity by Stevioside in Fructose-Rich Chow-Fed Rats." *Hormone and Metabolic Research* 37 (10): 610–16.

Chaudhary, D. P., R. Sharma, and D. D. Bansal. 2010. "Implications of Magnesium Deficiency in Type 2 Diabetes: A Review." *Biological Trace Element Research* 134 (2): 119–29.

Chen, J. Q., T. R. Brown, and J. Russo. 2009. "Regulation of Energy Metabolism Pathways by Estrogens and Estrogenic Chemicals and Potential Implications in Obesity Associated with Increased Exposure to Endocrine Disruptors." *Biochimica et Biophysica Acta* 1793 (7): 1128–43.

Chen, R. C., M. S. Lee, Y. H. Chang, and M. L. Wahlqvist. 2012. "Cooking Frequency May Enhance Survival in Taiwanese Elderly." *Public Health Nutrition* 15 (7): 1142–49.

Chen, Y. W., C. Y. Yang, C. F. Huang, D. Z. Hung, Y. M. Leung, and S. H. Liu. 2009. "Heavy Metals, Islet Function and Diabetes Development." *Islets* 1 (3): 169–76.

Cho, K. M., R. K. Math, S. M. Islam, W. J. Lim, S. Y. Hong, J. M. Kim, M. G. Yun, J. J. Cho, and H. D. Yun. 2009. "Biodegradation of Chlorpyrifos by Lactic Acid Bacteria During Kimchi Fermentation." *Journal of Agricultural and Food Chemistry* 57 (5): 1882–89.

Church, T. S., S. N. Blair, S. Cocreham, N. Johannsen, W. Johnson, K. Kramer, et al. 2010. "Effects of Aerobic and Resistance Training on Hemoglobin A1c Levels in Patients with Type 2 Diabetes: A Randomized Controlled Trial." *Journal of the American Medical Association* 304 (20): 2253–62.

Cohen, A. E., and C. S. Johnston. 2011. "Almond Ingestion at Mealtime Reduces Postprandial Glycemia and Chronic Ingestion Reduces Hemoglobin A(1c) in Individuals with Well-Controlled Type 2 Diabetes Mellitus." *Metabolism* 60 (9): 1312–17.

Craft, L. L., T. W. Zderic, S. M. Gapstur, E. H. Vaniterson, D. M. Thomas, J. Siddique, and M. T. Hamilton. 2012. "Evidence That Women Meeting Physical Activity Guidelines Do Not Sit Less: An Observational Inclinometry Study." *International Journal of Behavioral Nutrition and Physical Activity* 9: 122.

Crinnion, W. J. 2000. "Environmental Medicine, Part 4: Pesticides. Biologically Persistent and Ubiquitous Toxins." *Alternative Medicine Review* 5 (5): 432–47.

———. 2010. *Clean, Green, and Lean: Get Rid of the Toxins That Make You Fat.* Hoboken, NJ: John Wiley and Sons.

———. 2011. "Sauna as a Valuable Clinical Tool for Cardiovascular, Autoimmune, Toxicant-Induced and Other Chronic Health Problems." *Alternative Medicine Review* 16 (3): 215–25.

Dahlgren, J., M. Cecchini, H. Takhar, and O. Paepke. 2007. "Persistent Organic Pollutants in 9/11 World Trade Center Rescue Workers: Reduction Following Detoxification." *Chemosphere* 69 (8): 1320–25.

Daley, C. A., A. Abbott, P. S. Doyle, G. A. Nader, and S. Larson. 2010. "A Review of Fatty Acid Profiles and Antioxidant Content in Grass-Fed and Grain-Fed Beef." *Nutrition Journal* 9:10.

Danby, F. W. 2010. "Nutrition and Aging Skin: Sugar and Glycation." *Clinical Dermatology* 28 (4): 409–11.

Dannenberg, A. J., and E. K. Yang. 1992. "Effect of Dietary Lipids on Levels of UDP-Glucuronosyltransferase in Liver." *Biochemical Pharmacology* 44 (2): 335–40.

Dean, A., and J. Armstrong. 2009. "Genetically Modified Foods." Reviewed and approved by the American Academy of Environmental Medicine on May 8. http://www.aaemonline.org/gmopost.html.

Dorana, C. M., L. Valenti, M. Robinson, H. Britt, and R. P. Mattick. 2006. "Smoking Status of Australian General Practice Patients and Their Attempts to Quit." *Addictive Behaviors* 31 (5): 758–66.

Eliasson, B., M. R. Taskinen, and U. Smith. 1996. "Long-Term Use of Nicotine Gum Is Associated with Hyperinsulinemia and Insulin Resistance." *Circulation* 94 (5): 878–81.

EPA (Environmental Protection Agency). 2008. "2006 Inventory Update Reporting: Data Summary." EPA 740S08001. http://www.epa.gov/hpv /pubs/general/hazchem.htm

———. 2012a. "An Introduction to Indoor Air Quality: Volatile Organic Compounds." http://www.epa.gov/iaq/voc.html.

———. 2012b. "2000-2001 Pesticide Market Estimates: Usage." http://www .epa.gov/pesticides/pestsales/01pestsales/usage2001.htm.

———. 2012c. "The Inside Story: A Guide to Indoor Air Quality." http:// www.epa.gov/iaq/pubs/insidestory.html.

———. 2013. "Long-Chain Perfluorinated Chemicals (PFCs) Action Plan Summary." http://www.epa.gov/opptintr/existingchemicals/pubs/action-plans/pfcs.html.

Epstein, S. S. 1990. "The Chemical Jungle: Today's Beef Industry." *International Journal of Health Services* 20 (2): 277–80.

EWG (Environmental Working Group). 2008. "Bottled Water Quality Investigation: Ten Major Brands, Thirty-Eight Pollutants." http://www .worldcat.org/arcviewer/2/WCA/2009/11/16/H1258409800257 /viewer/file2.html.

———. 2009a. "Over 300 Pollutants in US Tap Water." http://www.ewg.org/ tap-water/.

———. 2009b. "Pollution in Minority Newborns: BPA and Other Cord Blood Pollutants." http://www.ewg.org/research/minority-cord-blood -report/bpa-and-other-cord-blood-pollutants.

———. 2011. "Why This Matters: Cosmetics and Your Health." http://www .ewg.org/skindeep/2011/04/12/why-this-matters/.

———. 2013. "EWG's 2013 Shopper's Guide to Pesticides in Produce." http://www.ewg.org/foodnews/list.php.

Fantuzzi, G. 2005. "Adipose Tissue, Adipokines, and Inflammation." *Journal of Allergy and Clinical Immunology* 115 (5): 911–19.

Felton, C. V., D. Crook, M. J. Davies, and M. F. Oliver. 1994. "Dietary Polyunsaturated Fatty Acids and Composition of Human Aortic Plaques." *Lancet* 344 (8931): 1195–96.

Fischer-Posovszky, P., V. Kukulus, M. A. Zulet, K. M. Debatin, and M. Wabitsch. 2007. "Conjugated Linoleic Acids Promote Human Fat Cell Apoptosis." *Hormone and Metabolic Research* 39 (3): 186–91.

Flachs, P., M. Rossmeisl, M. Bryhn, and J. Kopecky. 2009. "Cellular and Molecular Effects of N-3 Polyunsaturated Fatty Acids on Adipose Tissue Biology and Metabolism." *Clinical Science* (London) 116 (1): 1–16.

Flora, S. J. S., and V. Pachauri. 2010. "Chelation in Metal Intoxication." *International Journal of Environmental Research and Public Health* 7 (7): 2745–88.

Fowke, J. H., J. D. Morrow, S. Motley, R. M. Bostick, and R. M. Ness. 2006. "Brassica Vegetable Consumption Reduces Urinary F2-Isoprostane Levels Independent of Micronutrient Intake." *Carcinogenesis* 27 (10): 2096–102.

Gerster, H. 1998. "Can Adults Adequately Convert Alpha-Linolenic Acid (18:3n-3) to Eicosapentaenoic Acid (20:5n-3) and Docosahexaenoic Acid (22:6n-3)?" *International Journal of Vitamin and Nutrition Research* 68 (3): 159–73.

Ghannam, N., M Kingston, I. A. Al-Meshaal, M. Tariq, N. S. Parman, and N. Woodhouse. 1986. "The Antidiabetic Activity of Aloes: Preliminary Clinical and Experimental Observations." *Hormone Research* 24 (4): 288–94.

Godfrey, K. M., H. M. Inskip, and M. A. Hanson. 2011. "The Long-Term Effects of Prenatal Development on Growth and Metabolism." *Seminars in Reproductive Medicine* 29 (3): 257–65.

Gomes, E. C., J. E. Allgrove, G. Florida-James, and V. Stone. 2011. "Effect of Vitamin Supplementation on Lung Injury and Running Performance in a Hot, Humid, and Ozone-Polluted Environment." *Scandinavian Journal of Medicine and Science in Sports* 21 (6): e452–60.

Gooley, J. J., K. Chamberlain, K. A. Smith, S. B. Khalsa, S. M. Rajaratnam, E. Van Reen, J. M. Zeitzer, C. A. Czeisler, and S. W. Lockley. 2011. "Exposure to Room Light Before Bedtime Suppresses Melatonin Onset and Shortens Melatonin Duration in Humans." *Journal of Clinical Endocrinology and Metabolism* 96 (3): E463–72.

Goto, K., N. Ishii, K. Kurokawa, and K. Takamatsu. 2007. "Attenuated Growth Hormone Response to Resistance Exercise with Prior Sprint Exercise." *Medicine and Science in Sports and Exercise* 39 (1):108–15.

Grassi, D., C. Lippi, S. Necozione, G.Desideri, and C. Ferri. 2005. "Short-Term Administration of Dark Chocolate Is Followed by a Significant Increase in Insulin Sensitivity and a Decrease in Blood Pressure in Healthy Persons." *American Journal of Clinical Nutrition* 81(3): 611–14.

Graudal, N. A., T. Hubeck-Graudal, and G. Jurgens. 2011. "Effects of Low Sodium Diet Versus High Sodium Diet on Blood Pressure, Renin, Aldosterone, Catecholamines, Cholesterol, and Triglyceride." *Cochrane Database of Systematic Reviews* 11: CD004022.

Gregersen S., P. B. Jeppesen, J. J. Holst, and K. Hermansen. 2004. "Antihyperglycemic Effects of Stevioside in Type 2 Diabetic Subjects." *Metabolism* 53 (1): 73–76.

Grøntved, A., E. B. Rimm, W. C. Willett, L. B. Andersen, and F. B. Hu. 2012. "A Prospective Study of Weight Training and Risk of Type 2

Diabetes Mellitus in Men." *Archives of Internal Medicine* 172 (17): 1306–12.

Harvey, C., and P. W. French. 2000. "Effects on Protein Kinase C and Gene Expression in a Human Mast Cell Line, HMC-1, Following Microwave Exposure." *Cell Biology International* 23 (11): 739–48.

Havas, M. 2008. "Dirty Electricity Elevates Blood Sugar Among Electrically Sensitive Diabetics and May Explain Brittle Diabetes." *Electromagnetic Biology and Medicine* 27 (2):135–46.

Hegde, S. V., P. Adhikari, S. Kotian, V. J. Pinto, S. D'Souza, and V. D'Souza. 2011. "Effect of 3-Month Yoga on Oxidative Stress in Type 2 Diabetes with or Without Complications: A Controlled Clinical Trial." *Diabetes Care* 34 (10): 2208–10.

Holt-Lunstad, J., T. B. Smith, and J. B. Layton. 2010. "Social Relationships and Mortality Risk: A Meta-Analytic Review." *PLoS Medicine* 7 (7): e1000316.

Hong, Y. C., E. Y. Park, M. S. Park. J. A. Ko, S. Y. Oh, H. Kim, K. H. Lee, J. H. Leem, and E. H. Ha. 2009. "Community Level Exposure to Chemicals and Oxidative Stress in Adult Population." *Toxicology Letters* 184 (2): 139–44.

Hoppe, C., C. Mølgaard, A. Vaag, V. Barkholt, and K. F. Michaelsen. 2005. "High Intakes of Milk, but Not Meat, Increase S-Insulin and Insulin Resistance in Eight-Year-Old Boys." *European Journal of Clinical Nutrition* 59 (3): 393–98.

Hue, O., J. Marcotte, F. Berrigan, M. Simoneau, J. Doré, P. Marceau P., S. Marceau, A. Tremblay, and N. Teasdale. 2007. "Plasma Concentration of Organochlorine Compounds Is Associated with Age and Not Obesity." *Chemosphere* 67 (7): 1463–67.

Huebschmann, A. G., W. M. Kohrt, and J. G. Regensteiner. 2011. "Exercise Attenuates the Premature Cardiovascular Aging Effects of Type 2 Diabetes Mellitus." *Vascular Medicine* 16 (5): 378–90.

Innes, K. E., and H. K. Vincent. 2007. "The Influence of Yoga-Based Programs on Risk Profiles in Adults with Type 2 Diabetes Mellitus: A Systematic Review." *Evidence-Based Complementary and Alternative Medicine* 4 (4): 469–86.

International Bottled Water Association. 2008. "Bottled Water: More Than Just a Story About Sales Growth." http://www.bottledwater.org/content /bottled-water-more-just-story-about-sales-growth.

Isolauri, E. 2001. "Probiotics in Human Disease." *American Journal of Clinical Nutrition* 73 (6): 1142S–1146S.

Jee, S. H., H. Ohrr, J. W. Sull, J. E. Yun, M. Ji, and J. M. Samet. 2005. "Fasting Serum Glucose Level and Cancer Risk in Korean Men and Women." *Journal of the American Medical Association* 293 (2): 194–202.

Johnston, C. S., I. Steplewska, C. A. Long, L. N. Harris, and R. H. Ryals. 2010. "Examination of the Antiglycemic Properties of Vinegar in Healthy Adults." *Annals of Nutrition and Metabolism* 56 (1): 74–79.

Kanter, M., O. Coskun, and A. Gurel. 2005. "Effect of Black Cumin (Nigella Sativa) on Cadmium-Induced Oxidative Stress in the Blood of Rats." *Biological Trace Element Research* 107 (3): 277–87.

Keyse, S. M., and R. M. Tyrrell. 1987. "Both Near Ultraviolet Radiation and the Oxidizing Agent Hydrogen Peroxide Induce a 32-Kda Stress Protein in Normal Human Skin Fibroblasts." *Journal of Biological Chemistry* 262 (30): 14821–25.

Kim, K. J., M. J. Kil, J. S. Song, and E. H. Yoo. 2008. "Efficiency of Volatile Formaldehyde Removal by Indoor Plants: Contribution of Aerial Plant Parts Versus the Root Zone." *Journal of the American Society for Horticulture Science* 133 (4): 521–26.

King D. E., A. G. Mainous 3rd, M. E. Geesey, and R. F. Woolson. 2005. "Dietary Magnesium and C-Reactive Protein Levels." *Journal of the American College of Nutrition* 24 (3): 166–71.

Knowler, W. C., E. Barrett-Connor, S. E. Fowler, R. F. Hamman, J. M. Lachin, E. A. Walker, and D. M. Nathan. 2002. "Reduction in the Incidence of Type 2 Diabetes with Lifestyle Intervention or Metformin." *New England Journal of Medicine* 346 (6): 393–403.

Knutson, K. L., and E. Van Cauter. 2008. "Associations Between Sleep Loss and Increased Risk of Obesity and Diabetes." *Annals of the New York Academy of Sciences* 1129: 287–304.

Kolpin, D. W., E. T. Furlong, M. T. Meyer, E. M. Thurman, S. D. Zaugg, L. B. Barber, and H. Buxton. 2002. "Pharmaceuticals, Hormones, and Other Organic Wastewater Contaminants in US Streams, 1999–2000: A National Reconnaissance." *Environmental Science and Technology* 36 (6):1202–11.

Krogsbøll, L. T., K. J. Jørgensen, C. Grønhøj Larsen, and P. C. Gøtzsche. 2012. "General Health Checks in Adults for Reducing Morbidity and Mortality from Disease." *Cochrane Database of Systematic Reviews* 10: CD009009. doi: 10.1002/14651858.CD009009.pub2.

Lee, A. T., and A. Cerami. 1987. "The Formation of Reactive Intermediate(s) of Glucose 6-Phosphate and Lysine Capable of Rapidly Reacting with DNA." *Mutation Research* 179 (2): 151–58.

Lee, D. H., M. W. Steffes, A. Sjödin, R. S. Jones, L. L. Needham, and D. R. Jacobs Jr. 2010. "Low Dose of Some Persistent Organic Pollutants Predicts Type 2 Diabetes: A Nested Case-Control Study." *Environmental Health Perspectives* 118 (9): 1235–42.

Liang Y., V. Maier, G. Steinbach, L. Lalić, and E. F. Pfeiffer. 1987. "The Effect of Artificial Sweetener on Insulin Secretion. II. Stimulation of

Insulin Release from Isolated Rat Islets by Acesulfame K (In Vitro Experiments)." *Hormone and Metabolic Research* 19 (7): 285–89.

Lii, C. K., K. L. Liu, Y. P. Cheng, A. H. Lin, H. W. Chen, and C. W. Tsai. 2010. "Sulforaphane and Alpha-Lipoic Acid Upregulate the Expression of the Pi Class of Glutathione S-Transferase through C-Jun and Nrf2 Activation." *Journal of Nutrition* 140 (5): 885–92.

Lim, G. P., T. Chu, F. Yang, W. Beech, S. A. Frautschy, and G. M. Cole. 2001. "The Curry Spice Curcumin Reduces Oxidative Damage and Amyloid Pathology in an Alzheimer Transgenic Mouse." *Journal of Neuroscience* 21(21): 8370–77.

Lin C. Y., P. C. Chen, Y. C. Lin, and L.Y. Lin. 2009. "Association Among Serum Perfluoroalkyl Chemicals, Glucose Homeostasis, and Metabolic Syndrome in Adolescents and Adults." *Diabetes Care* 32 (4): 702–7.

Liska, D. J., and J. S. Bland. 2002. "Emerging Clinical Science of Bifunctional Support for Detoxification." *Townsend Letter for Doctors and Patients* 231: 42–46.

Lo, H. C., and S. P. Wasser. 2011. "Medicinal Mushrooms for Glycemic Control in Diabetes Mellitus: History, Current Status, Future Perspectives, and Unsolved Problems (Review)." *International Journal of Medicinal Mushrooms* 13 (5): 401–26.

Madkor, H. R., S. W. Mansour, and G. Ramadan. 2011. "Modulatory Effects of Garlic, Ginger, Turmeric and Their Mixture on Hyperglycaemia, Dyslipidaemia and Oxidative Stress in Streptozotocin-Nicotinamide Diabetic Rats." *British Journal of Nutrition* 105 (8): 1210–17.

Mandel, S., T. Amit, L. Reznichenko, O. Weinreb, and M. B. Youdim. 2006. "Green Tea Catechins as Brain-Permeable, Natural Iron Chelators-Antioxidants for the Treatment of Neurodegenerative Disorders." *Molecular Nutrition and Food Research* 50 (2): 229–34.

Mani, U. V., I. Mani, M. Biswas, and S. N. Kumar. 2011. "An Open-Label Study on the Effect of Flax Seed Powder (Linum usitatissimum) Supplementation in the Management of Diabetes Mellitus." *Journal of Dietary Supplements.* 8 (3): 257–65.

Markus, C. R., B. Olivier, G. E. Panhuysen, J. Van Der Gugten, M. S. Alles, A. Tuiten, H. G. Westenberg, D. Fekkes, H. F. Koppeschaar, and E. E. Haan. 2000. "The Bovine Protein Alpha-Lactalbumin Increases the Plasma Ratio of Tryptophan to the Other Large Neutral Amino Acids, and in Vulnerable Subjects Raises Brain Serotonin Activity, Reduces Cortisol Concentration, and Improves Mood Under Stress." *American Journal of Clinical Nutrition* 71 (6): 1536–44.

Marnewick, J. L., E. Joubert, P. Swart, F. Van Der Westhuizen, and W. C. Gelderblom. 2003. "Modulation of Hepatic Drug Metabolizing Enzymes and Oxidative Status by Rooibos (Aspalathus linearis) and Honeybush

(Cyclopia intermedia), Green and Black (Camellia sinensis) Teas in Rats." *Journal of Agricultural and Food Chemistry* 51 (27): 8113–19.

McAfee, A. J., E. M. McSorley, G. J. Cuskelly, A. M. Fearon, B. W. Moss, J. A. Beattie, J. M. Wallace, M. P. Bonham, and J. J. Strain. 2011. "Red Meat from Animals Offered a Grass Diet Increases Plasma and Platelet N-3 PUFA in Healthy Consumers." *British Journal of Nutrition*. 2011 105 (1): 80–89.

Mead, M. N. 2008. "Benefits of Sunlight: A Bright Spot for Human Health." *Environmental Health Perspectives* 116 (4): A160–67.

Mekary, R. A., E. Giovannucci, W. C. Willett, R. M. van Dam, and F. B. Hu. 2012. "Eating Patterns and Type 2 Diabetes Risk in Men: Breakfast Omission, Eating Frequency, and Snacking." *American Journal of Clinical Nutrition* 95 (5) :1182–89.

Mitri, J., B. Dawson-Hughes, F. B. Hu, and A. G. Pittas. 2011. "Effects of Vitamin D and Calcium Supplementation on Pancreatic Cell Function, Insulin Sensitivity, and Glycemia in Adults at High Risk of Diabetes: The Calcium and Vitamin D for Diabetes Mellitus (Caddm) Randomized Controlled Trial." *American Journal of Clinical Nutrition* 94 (2): 486–94.

Morita, K., T. Matsueda, and T. Iida. 1999. "Effect of Green Vegetable on Digestive Tract Absorption of Polychlorinated Dibenzo-P-Dioxins and Polychlorinated Dibenzofurans in Rats." Article in Japanese. *Fukuoka Igaku Zasshi* 90 (5): 171–83.

Na, H. K., and Y. J. Surh. 2008. "Modulation of Nrf2-Mediated Antioxidant and Detoxifying Enzyme Induction by the Green Tea Polyphenol EGCG." *Food and Chemical Toxicology* 46 (4):1271–78.

Nagabhushan, M., and S. V. Bhide. 1992. "Curcumin as an Inhibitor of Cancer." *Journal of the American College of Nutrition* 11 (2): 192–98.

Nagendra, R. P., N. Maruthai, and B. M. Kutty1. 2012. "Meditation and Its Regulatory Role on Sleep." *Frontiers in Neurology* 3: 54.

Netherwood T., S. M. Martín-Orúe, A. G. O'Donnell, S. Gockling, J. Graham, J. C. Mathers, and H. J. Gilbert. 2004. "Assessing the Survival of Transgenic Plant DNA in the Human Gastrointestinal Tract." *Nature Biotechnology* 22 (2): 204–9.

Nick, G. L. 2002. "Detoxification Properties of Low-Dose Phytochemical Complexes Found within Select Vegetables." *Journal of the American Nutraceutical Association* 5 (4): 34–44.

NIDDK (National Institute of Diabetes and Digestive and Kidney Diseases). 2012. Diagnosis of Diabetes and Prediabetes. National Institutes of Health Publication No. 12-4642. http://www.diabetes.niddk.nih.gov /dm/pubs/diagnosis.

O'Hara, A. M., and F. Shanahan. 2006. "The Gut Flora as a Forgotten Organ." *EMBO Reports* 7 (7): 688–93.

Ohtsuka, Y., N. Yabunaka, and S. Takayama. 1998. "Shinrin-Yoku (Forest-Air Bathing and Walking) Effectively Decreases Blood Glucose Levels in Diabetic Patients." *International Journal of Biometeorology* 41 (3): 125–27.

Ornish D., M. J. Magbanua, G. Weidner, V. Weinberg, C. Kemp, C. Green, et al. 2008. "Changes in Prostate Gene Expression in Men Undergoing an Intensive Nutrition and Lifestyle Intervention." *Proceedings of the National Acadeny of Sciences of the United States of America* 105(24):8369–74.

Omura, Y., and S. L. Beckman. 1995. "Role of Mercury (Hg) in Resistant Infections and Effective Treatment of Chlamydia Trachomatis and Herpes Family Viral Infections (and Potential Treatment for Cancer) by Removing Localized Hg Deposits with Chinese Parsley and Delivering Effective Antibiotics Using Various Drug Uptake Enhancement Methods." *Acupuncture and Electrotherapeutics Research* 20 (3–4): 195–229.

Ozercan, I. H., A. F. Dagli, B. Ustundag, M. R. Ozercan, I. H. Bahcecioglu, H. Celik, M. Yalniz, O. K. Poyrazoglu, and H. Ataseven. 2006. "Does Instant Coffee Prevent Acute Liver Injury Induced by Carbon Tetrachloride (Ccl(4))?" *Hepatology Research* 35 (3): 163–68.

Papinchak, H. L., E. J. Holcomb, T. O. Best, and D. R. Decoteau. 2009. "Effectiveness of Houseplants in Reducing the Indoor Air Pollutant Ozone." *HortTechnology* 19 (2): 286–90.

Pastors, J. G., P. W. Blaisdell, T. K. Balm, C. M. Asplin, and S. L. Pohl. 1991. "Psyllium Fiber Reduces Rise in Postprandial Glucose and Insulin Concentrations in Patients with Non-Insulin-Dependent Diabetes." *American Journal of Clinical Nutrition* 53 (6): 1431–35.

Persson, E., G. Graziani, R. Ferracane, V. Fogliano, and K. Skog. 2003. "Influence of Antioxidants in Virgin Olive Oil on the Formation of Heterocyclic Amines in Fried Beefburgers." *Food and Chemical Toxicology* 41 (11): 1587–97.

Phelps, J. 2008. "Dark Therapy for Bipolar Disorder Using Amber Lenses for Blue Light Blockade." *Medical Hypotheses* 70 (2): 224–29.

Poh, Z. X., and K. P. Goh. 2009. "A Current Update on the Use of Alpha Lipoic Acid in the Management of Type 2 Diabetes Mellitus." *Endocrine, Metabolic and Immune Disorders Drug Targets* 9 (4): 392–98.

Preuss, H. G., B. Echard, N. V. Perricone, D. Bagchi, T. Yasmin, and S. J. Stohs. 2008. "Comparing Metabolic Effects of Six Different Commercial Trivalent Chromium Compounds." *Journal of Inorganic Biochemistry* 102 (11): 1986–90.

Psaltopoulou, T., I. Ilias, and M. Alevizaki. 2010. "The Role of Diet and Lifestyle in Primary, Secondary, and Tertiary Diabetes Prevention: A Review of Meta-Analyses." *The Review of Diabetic Studies* 7 (1): 26–35.

Qin J., Y. Li, Z. Cai, S. Li, J. Zhu, F. Zhang, et al. 2012. "A Metagenome-Wide Association Study of Gut Microbiota in Type 2 Diabetes." *Nature* 490 (7418): 55–60.

Radzevičienė, L., and R. Ostrauskas. 2012. "Fast Eating and the Risk of Type 2 Diabetes Mellitus: A Case-Control Study." *Clinical Nutrition.* Published electronically July 5. http://www.clinicalnutritionjournal.com/article /S0261-5614(12)00136-7/fulltext.

Rafalson, L., R. P. Donahue, J. Dmochowski, K. Rejman, J. Dorn, and M. Trevisan. 2009. "Cigarette Smoking Is Associated with Conversion from Normoglycemia to Impaired Fasting Glucose: The Western New York Health Study." *Annals of Epidemiology* 19 (6): 365–71.

Rani, M. P., K. P. Padmakumari, B. Sankarikutty, O. L. Cherian, V. M. Nisha, and K. G. Raghu. 2011. "Inhibitory Potential of Ginger Extracts against Enzymes Linked to Type 2 Diabetes, Inflammation and Induced Oxidative Stress." *International Journal of Food Sciences and Nutrition* 62 (2):106–10.

Reis, J. P., D. von Mühlen, E. R. Miller 3rd, E. D. Michos, and L. J. Appel. 2009. "Vitamin D Status and Cardiometabolic Risk Factors in the United States Adolescent Population." *Pediatrics* 124 (3): e371–79.

Reuben, S. 2010. "Reducing Environmental Cancer Risk: What We Can Do Now." 2008–2009 Annual Report for the President's Cancer Panel, US Department of Health and Human Services. Submitted in April. http:// www.deainfo.nci.nih.gov/advisory/pcp/annualReports/pcp08-09rpt /PCP_Report_08-09_508.pdf.

Ropero, A. B., P. Alonso-Magdalena, E. García-García, C. Ripoll, E. Fuentes, and A. Nadal. 2008. "Bisphenol-A Disruption of the Endocrine Pancreas and Blood Glucose Homeostasis." *International Journal of Andrology* 31 (2): 194–200.

Rudel, R. A., D. E. Camann, J. D. Spengler, L. R. Korn, and J. G. Brody. 2003. "Phthalates, Alkylphenols, Pesticides, Polybrominated Diphenyl Ethers, and Other Endocrine-Disrupting Compounds in Indoor Air and Dust." *Environmental Science and Technology* 37 (20): 4543–53.

Rudel, R. A., J. M. Gray, C. L. Engel, T. W. Rawsthorne, R. E. Dodson, J. M. Ackerman, J. L. Nudelman, and J. G. Brody. 2011. "Food Packaging and Bisphenol A and Bis(2-Ethyhexyl) Phthalate Exposure: Findings from a Dietary Intervention." *Environmental Health Perspectives* 119 (7): 914–20.

Saito, M., Y. Hattori, and M. Eto. 2011. "Thorough Chewing Stimulates Postprandial Increases of Plasma GLP-1 and Peptide YY in Obese Subjects." Abstract presented at the European Association for the Study of Diabetes 47th Annual Meeting, Lisbon, September 13.

Salmerón, J., F. B. Hu, J. E. Manson, M. J. Stampfer, G. A. Colditz, E. B. Rimm, and W. C. Willett. 2001. "Dietary Fat Intake and Risk of Type 2

Diabetes in Women." *American Journal of Clinical Nutrition* 73 (6): 1019–26.

Sanchis-Gomar, F., J. L. Garcia-Gimenez, C. Perez-Quilis C., M. C. Gomez-Cabrera, F. V. Pallardo, and G. Lippi. 2012. "Physical Exercise as an Epigenetic Modulator: Eustress, the 'Positive Stress' as an Effector of Gene Expression." *Journal of Strength and Conditioning Research* 26 (12): 3469–72.

Sartorelli, D. S., R. Damião, R. Chaim, A. Hirai, S. G. Gimeno, and S. R. Ferreira; the Japanese-Brazilian Diabetes Study Group. 2010. "Dietary Omega-3 Fatty Acid and Omega-3: Omega-6 Fatty Acid Ratio Predict Improvement in Glucose Disturbances in Japanese Brazilians." *Nutrition* 26 (2): 184–91.

Scalbert, A., C. Manach, C. Morand, C. Rémésy, and L. Jiménez. 2005. "Dietary Polyphenols and the Prevention of Diseases." *Critical Reviews in Food Science and Nutrition* 45 (4): 287–306.

Serraino, I., L. Dugo, P. Dugo, L. Mondello, E. Mazzon, G. Dugo, A. P. Caputi, and S. Cuzzocrea. 2003. "Protective Effects of Cyanidin-3-O-Glucoside from Blackberry Extract Against Peroxynitrite-Induced Endothelial Dysfunction and Vascular Failure." *Life Sciences* 73 (9): 1097–114.

Shanahan, S., and L. Shanahan. 2009. *Deep Nutrition: Why Your Genes Need Traditional Food.* Lawai, Hawaii: Big Box Books.

Shay, K. P., R. F. Moreau, E. J. Smith, A. R. Smith, and T. M. Hagen. 2009. "Alpha-Lipoic Acid as a Dietary Supplement: Molecular Mechanisms and Therapeutic Potential." *Biochimica et Biophysica Acta* 1790 (10): 1149–60.

Shoba, G., D. Joy, T. Joseph, M. Majeed, R. Rajendran, and P. S. Srinivas. 1998. "Influence of Piperine on the Pharmacokinetics of Curcumin in Animals and Human Volunteers." *Planta Medica* 64 (4): 353–56.

Simopoulos, A. P. 2008. "The Importance of the Omega-6/Omega-3 Fatty Acid Ratio in Cardiovascular Disease and Other Chronic Diseases." *Experimental Biology and Medicine* 233 (6): 674–88.

Sinatra, S. 2007. *Reverse Heart Disease Now: Stop Deadly Cardiovascular Plaque Before It's Too Late.* Hoboken, NJ: John Wiley and Sons.

Singh, U., and I. Jialal. 2008. "Alpha-Lipoic Acid Supplementation and Diabetes." *Nutrition Reviews* 66 (11): 646–57.

Siri-Tarino, P. W., Q. Sun, F. B. Hu, and R. M. Krauss. 2010. "Meta-Analysis of Prospective Cohort Studies Evaluating the Association of Saturated Fat with Cardiovascular Disease." *American Journal of Clinical Nutrition* 91 (3): 535–46.

Sokal, K., and P. Sokal. 2011. "Earthing the Human Body Influences Physiologic Processes." *Journal of Alternative and Complementary Medicine* 17 (4): 301–8.

Sreelatha, S., and R. Inbavalli. 2012. "Antioxidant, Antihyperglycemic, and Antihyperlipidemic Effects of Coriandrum Sativum Leaf and Stem in Alloxan-Induced Diabetic Rats." *Journal of Food Science* 77 (7): T119–23.

Sreelatha, S., P. R. Padma, and M. Umadevi. 2009. "Protective Effects of Coriandrum Sativum Extracts on Carbon Tetrachloride-Induced Hepatotoxicity in Rats." *Food and Chemical Toxicology* 47 (4): 702–8.

Steptoe, A., and J. Wardle. 2005. "Positive Affect and Biological Function in Everyday Life." *Neurobiology of Aging* 26 (Suppl 1): 108–12.

Svensson, K., R. U. Hernández-Ramírez, A. Burguete-García, M. E. Cebrián, A. M. Calafat, L. L. Needham, L. Claudio, and L. López-Carrillo. 2011. "Phthalate Exposure Associated with Self-Reported Diabetes Among Mexican Women." *Environmental Research* 111 (6): 792–96.

Talanian, J. L., S. D. Galloway, G. J. Heigenhauser, A. Bonen, and L. L. Spriet. 2007. "Two Weeks of High-Intensity Aerobic Interval Training Increases the Capacity for Fat Oxidation During Exercise in Women." *Journal of Applied Psychology* 102 (4): 1439–47.

Tang, Y. Y. 2011. "Mechanism of Integrative Body-Mind Training." *Neuroscience Bulletin* 27 (6): 383–88.

Thomas, D. E., E. J. Elliott, and G. A. Naughton. 2006. "Exercise for Type 2 Diabetes Mellitus." *Cochrane Database of Systematic Reviews* (3): CD002968.

Tilgner, S. 1999. *Herbal Medicine from the Heart of the Earth*. Oregon: Wise Acres Press.

Tirosh, A., I. Shai, D. Tekes-Manova, E. Israeli, D. Pereg, T. Shochat, I. Kochba, A. Rudich; Israeli Diabetes Research Group. 2005. "Normal Fasting Plasma Glucose Levels and Type 2 Diabetes in Young Men." *New England Journal of Medicine* 353 (14): 1454–62.

Tweed, J. O., S. H. Hsia, K. Lutfy, and T. C. Friedman. 2012. "The Endocrine Effects of Nicotine and Cigarette Smoke." *Trends in Endocrinology and Metabolism* 23 (7): 334–42.

Ulicná, O., M. Greksák, O. Vancová, L. Zlatos, S. Galbavý, P. Bozek P., and M. Nakano. 2003. "Hepatoprotective Effect of Rooibos Tea (Aspalathus Linearis) on Ccl4-Induced Liver Damage in Rats." *Physiological Research* 52 (4): 461–66.

US Conference of Mayors. 2007. "Adopted Resolutions," from the US Conference of Mayors Seventy-Fifth Annual Meeting in June. http://www.usmayors.org/75thAnnualMeeting/resolutions_full.pdf.

USDA (United States Department of Agriculture). 2010. "Food Safety and Inspection Service National Residue Program for Cattle." Office of the Inspector General audit report 24601-08-KC, dated March 25. http://www.usda.gov/oig/webdocs/24601-08-KC.pdf.

———. 2011. "Annual Summary, Calendar Year 2009." Pesticide Data Program. http://www.ams.usda.gov/AMSv1.0/getfile?dDocName=STE LPRDC5091055

USFDA (United States Food and Drug Administration). 2012. "Food Allergies: What You Need to Know," last updated May 14. http://www.fda.gov/Food/ResourcesForYou/Consumers/ucm079311.htm.

Van Cauter, E., U. Holmback, K. Knutson, R. Leproult, A. Miller, A. Nedeltcheva, S. Pannain, P. Penev, E. Tasali, and K. Spiegel. 2007. "Impact of Sleep and Sleep Loss on Neuroendocrine and Metabolic Function." *Hormone Research* 67 (Suppl 1): 2–9.

Velussi, M., A. M. Cernigoi, A. De Monte, F. Dapas, C. Caffau, and M. Zilli. 1997. "Long-Term (12 Months) Treatment with an Anti-Oxidant Drug (Silymarin) Is Effective on Hyperinsulinemia, Exogenous Insulin Need and Malondialdehyde Levels in Cirrhotic Diabetic Patients." *Journal of Hepatology* 26 (4): 871–79.

Victor Antony Santiago, J., J. Jayachitra, M. Shenbagam, and N. Nalini. 2012. "Dietary D-Limonene Alleviates Insulin Resistance and Oxidative Stress-Induced Liver Injury in High-Fat Diet and L-NAME-Treated Rats." *European Journal of Nutrition* 51 (1): 57–68.

Villegas, R., Y. T. Gao, Q. Dai, G. Yang, H. Cai, H. Li, W. Zheng, and X. O. Shu. 2009. "Dietary Calcium and Magnesium Intakes and the Risk of Type 2 Diabetes: The Shanghai Women's Health Study." *American Journal of Clinical Nutrition* 89 (4): 1059–67.

Villegas, R., Y. B. Xiang, T. Elasy, H. L. Li, G. Yang, H. Cai, et al. 2011. "Fish, Shellfish, and Long-Chain N-3 Fatty Acid Consumption and Risk of Incident Type 2 Diabetes in Middle-Aged Chinese Men and Women." *American Journal of Clinical Nutrition* 94 (2): 543–51.

Volkow, N. D., D. Tomasi, G. J. Wang, P. Vaska, J. S. Fowler, F. Telang, S. Alexoff, J. Logan, and C. Wong. 2011. "Effects of Cell Phone Radiofrequency Signal Exposure on Brain Glucose Metabolism." *Journal of the American Medical Association* 305 (8): 808–13.

Vrieze A., E. Van Hood, F. Holleman, J. Salojärvi, and R. S. Kootte. 2012. Transfer of intestinal microbiota from lean donors increases insulin sensitivity in individuals with metabolic syndrome. *Gastroenterology* 143(4):913–6.e7.

Wang, C. H., C. C. Wang, and Y. H. Wei. 2010. "Mitochondrial Dysfunction in Insulin Insensitivity: Implication of Mitochondrial Role in Type 2 Diabetes." *Annals of the New York Academy of Sciences* 1201: 157–65.

Wang, S. L., P. C. Tsai, C. Y. Yang, and Y. L. Guo. 2008. "Increased Risk of Diabetes and Polychlorinated Biphenyls and Dioxins: A 24-Year Follow-Up Study of the Yucheng Cohort." *Diabetes Care* 31 (8): 1574–79.

Watson, N. F., K. P. Harden, D. Buchwald, M. V. Vitiello, A. I. Pack, D. S. Weigle, and J. Goldberg. 2012. "Sleep Duration and Body Mass Index in Twins: A Gene-Environment Interaction." *Sleep* 35 (5): 597–603.

Weinstein, J. 2006. *The Ethical Gourmet: How to Enjoy Great Food That Is Humanely Raised, Sustainable, Nonendangered, and That Replenishes the Earth.* New York: Random House.

Wellington, K., and B. Jarvis. 2001. "Silymarin: A Review of Its Clinical Properties in the Management of Hepatic Disorders." *BioDrugs* 15 (7): 465–89.

Westcott, W. L. 2012. "Resistance Training Is Medicine: Effects of Strength Training on Health." *Current Sports Medicine Reports* 11 (4): 209–16.

Wing, R. R., and the Look AHEAD Research Group. 2010. "Long-Term Effects of a Lifestyle Intervention on Weight and Cardiovascular Risk Factors in Individuals with Type 2 Diabetes Mellitus: Four-Year Results of the Look AHEAD Trial." *Archives of Internal Medicine* 170 (17): 1566–75.

World Health Organization. 2010. "Dioxins and Their Effects on Human Health." Fact Sheet No. 225. http://www.who.int/mediacentre/fact sheets/fs225/en/.

Yoo, M. H., Y. J. Kwon, and K. C. Son. 2006. "Efficacy of Indoor Plants for the Removal of Single and Mixed Volatile Organic Pollutants and Physiological Effects of the Volatiles on the Plants." *Journal of the American Society for Horticulture Science* 131 (4): 452–58.

Yuan, S.Y., C. Liu, C. S. Liao, and B. V. Chang. 2002. "Occurrence and Microbial Degradation of Phthalate Esters in Taiwan River Sediments." *Chemosphere* 49 (10):1295–99.

Sarah Cimperman, ND, is a naturopathic physician and an expert in natural medicine. In her private practice in New York City she focuses on nutrition, detoxification, and chronic illnesses including prediabetes. Her articles and expertise have been featured on Fox News and in *Natural Health* magazine, *Whole Living* magazine, and the *Well Being Journal*. Cimperman also writes about healthy eating and posts original recipes on her blog, *The Naturopathic Gourmet*. For more information, visit drsarahcimperman.com.

Foreword writer **Walter J. Crinnion, ND**, received his degree in naturopathic medicine from Bastyr University in Seattle, WA. He has published several articles in peer-reviewed journals on the topic of environmental overload. Crinnion has served on the board of directors at the American Association of Naturopathic Physicians and on the adjunct faculty of Bastyr University, the National College of Naturopathic Medicine in Portland, OR, and the University of Bridgeport College of Naturopathic Medicine in Bridgeport, CT. He is a professor at the Southwest College of Naturopathic Medicine in Tempe, AZ, and the chair of their environmental medicine department. In 2001 he appeared three times with Barbara Walters on ABC's *The View*. His first book, *Clean, Green, and Lean* was published by Wiley and Sons in 2009.

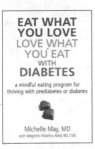
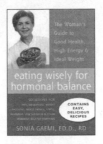
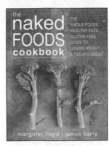
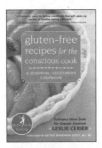
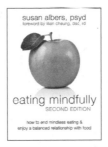
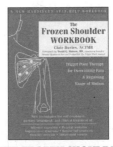